NURSING 101

A Comprehensive Guide to Help You Excel in Your Nursing Career

by Lorraine Voltaire

Disclaimer

This book is provided for general informational purposes only. The author has made every effort to ensure the content's accuracy and reliability; however, no guarantees are made regarding its completeness or applicability. Readers should seek professional advice tailored to their specific needs. The author and publisher disclaim any liability for any loss or harm incurred from the use or reliance on the information presented. All content is used at the reader's discretion and risk. The views expressed in this book are those of the author and do not necessarily reflect any affiliated organizations. No part of this publication may be reproduced without prior written consent, except brief quotations for reviews.

TABLE OF CONTENTS

INTRODUCTION

Welcome to the Profession: The Role of Nurses in Healthcare

Congratulations, and welcome to one of the most rewarding and impactful professions in the world—nursing! You've worked incredibly hard to get here, from memorizing pharmacology terms to surviving clinical rotations, and now you're stepping into a career that will change lives—both your patients' and your own.

As a nurse, you're not just providing care; you're an advocate, a teacher, and a leader. You'll be the person who notices subtle changes in a patient's condition and takes action. You'll be the reassuring presence for a family facing uncertainty. You'll bring knowledge, compassion, and skill to every interaction.

The role of a nurse is central to healthcare. Doctors rely on nurses to carry out care plans and report critical updates. Patients depend on you to be their voice when they can't speak for themselves. And your fellow nurses will look to you for teamwork and support. You are truly the backbone of healthcare, and while the journey ahead will be challenging, it will also be immensely fulfilling.

Transitioning from Nursing Student to Practicing Nurse

The transition from student to practicing nurse can feel overwhelming at first. Let's face it—textbooks and simulations can only prepare you so much. The first time you have a real patient relying on you, it's easy to second-guess yourself. That's normal! You're not alone in feeling that way.

Think of this phase as a steep learning curve. You're moving from theory to practice, from hypothetical cases to real-life patients with unique needs. It's okay to feel nervous—that's a sign that you care deeply about doing a good job.

As you enter the workplace, you'll quickly realize that nursing isn't just about knowing what to do; it's also about how you do it. Time management, communication, critical thinking, and teamwork will become just as important as clinical knowledge. The good news? You don't have to be perfect right away. Nursing is a journey, not a destination. Give yourself grace as you grow into your role.

Remember, you're not expected to know everything on Day 1. Lean on your colleagues, ask questions, and take every opportunity to learn. The nurses who thrive are the ones who never stop growing.

Why Avoiding Common Mistakes is Crucial for Success

Let's talk about something that isn't always emphasized in nursing school: mistakes. Everyone makes them. It's part of being human and part of learning. However, in healthcare, mistakes can have serious consequences—for your patients, your colleagues, and your career.

The good news is that many mistakes are avoidable if you know what to watch out for. That's what this book is all about. By learning from the missteps of others, you can set yourself up for success and provide the safest, most effective care possible.

Here's why avoiding common mistakes is so critical:

- **Patient Safety:** As a nurse, your primary responsibility is to keep your patients safe. Errors like giving the wrong medication or failing to recognize a change in a patient's condition can have life-threatening consequences. Avoiding these mistakes isn't just about following rules—it's about protecting the people who trust you with their care.
- **Professional Reputation:** Nursing is a team sport, and your colleagues need to trust you. Consistently making avoidable errors can damage your reputation and make it harder to build strong working relationships.
- **Personal Growth:** Making mistakes is part of learning, but repeating the same ones is a sign that something needs to change. By being proactive and mindful, you'll grow into a confident, competent nurse who others can rely on.

This book isn't here to scare you—it's here to empower you. By understanding common pitfalls and how to avoid them, you'll feel more confident stepping into your new role. Think of it as a roadmap for navigating the challenges of nursing with grace and resilience.

So, take a deep breath, and let's dive in. You've got this!

Chapter **One**

BUILDING Confidence

Starting your journey as a nurse is both exhilarating and intimidating. You're stepping into a world where you're no longer the student in the background—you're now a critical part of the team. That's a big responsibility! But don't worry; no one expects you to know everything on day one. What's more important than knowing it all is your willingness to learn, grow, and lean into the process. This chapter is all about how to build your confidence, sharpen your skills, and set yourself up for long-term success in your nursing career.

The Importance of Continuous Learning & Skill Improvement

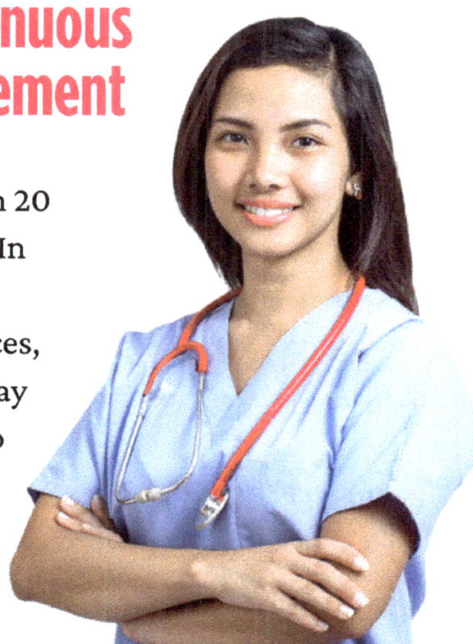

Here's a little secret: even nurses with 20 years of experience are still learning. In healthcare, change is constant. New research emerges, technology advances, and best practices evolve. The best way to stay confident in your abilities is to keep learning.

As a new nurse, you'll find that some things come naturally—maybe you're great at connecting with patients, or you've got a knack for staying organized during a busy shift. But there will be other areas that feel challenging, and that's okay. Use every day as an opportunity to sharpen your skills. Ask questions, take notes, and don't be afraid to admit when you don't know something.

Many hospitals and healthcare organizations offer ongoing training programs, workshops, and certifications. Sign up for these opportunities when you can. They're not just good for your resume—they're also a fantastic way to boost your competence and confidence.

Pro Tip: Keep a small notebook or an app on your phone where you jot down things you've learned or topics you need to review later. Over time, this collection of notes will become a treasure trove of knowledge that you can rely on.

Embracing Mentorship & Finding a Trusted Mentor

No nurse succeeds alone. One of the best things you can do as a new nurse is to find a mentor—someone who's been in your shoes and knows the ropes. A good mentor will guide you, support you, and help you navigate the challenges of your first few years.

Look for someone who has the qualities you admire. Are they calm under pressure? Do they communicate well with patients and families? Do they seem to genuinely enjoy what they do? Don't hesitate to ask if they'd be willing to mentor you. Most experienced nurses remember what it was like to be new and are happy to help.

Your mentor doesn't have to be just one person. Maybe one nurse helps you with clinical skills while another guides you on time management or patient communication. The more relationships you build, the stronger your support system will be.

Pro Tip: Mentorship isn't a one-way street. Show your gratitude by being respectful of their time and genuinely applying what they teach you.

Knowing Your Resources: Policies, Procedures, and Manuals

When you're feeling unsure about how to handle a situation, your resources are your best friend. Every facility has policies, procedures, and manuals designed to guide you in providing safe and effective care. These resources aren't just there for decoration—they're there to help you.

For example, if you're administering a medication you're unfamiliar with or performing a procedure you haven't done before, don't just wing it. Take a moment to consult the relevant guidelines. Your patients' safety depends on your willingness to pause, double-check, and follow best practices.

Many facilities now have digital platforms or apps that make it easy to access this information on the go. Familiarize yourself with these tools early on so you know where to find answers when you need them.

Pro Tip: During your orientation, take notes on where to find critical resources like drug guides, emergency protocols, or infection control procedures. Knowing where to look can save valuable time in high-pressure situations.

Building Relationships with the Healthcare Team

One of the most valuable lessons you'll learn early in your career is that nursing is a team sport. You're not working in isolation—you're part of a larger group that includes doctors, respiratory therapists, physical therapists, social workers, and more. Building strong relationships with your colleagues will make your job easier and more enjoyable.

Start by showing respect and a willingness to collaborate. Simple things like introducing yourself, offering to help when you can, and saying thank you go a long way. When everyone on the team feels supported, patient care improves, and the work environment becomes more positive.

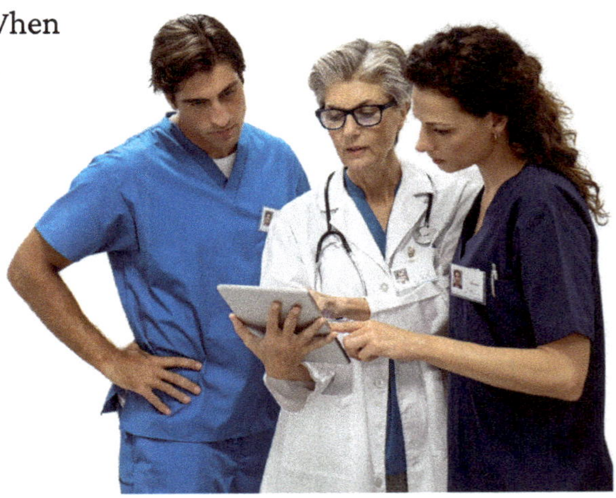

Communication is key. Whether you're handing off a patient to the next shift, discussing a care plan with a physician, or coordinating with other departments, clear and concise communication is essential. Don't be afraid to speak up if something doesn't seem right or if you need clarification.

Pro Tip: Build relationships with people outside your immediate team, too. The unit secretary, housekeeping staff, and dietary team all play critical roles in patient care. A little kindness and teamwork can create a stronger, more cohesive work environment.

Final Thoughts on Building Confidence and Competence

Confidence doesn't happen overnight—it's something you build over time through practice, learning, and connection. Remember, every seasoned nurse you admire was once in your shoes. They made mistakes, learned from them, and grew stronger because of it.

Take it one day at a time, embrace the process, and don't hesitate to lean on your resources and your team. Nursing is a journey, and you're just getting started. You've got this!

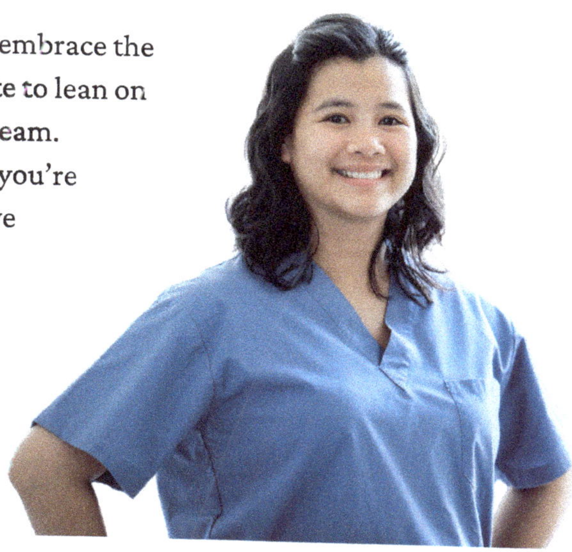

Chapter **Two**

EFFECTIVE Time Management

As a new nurse, you'll quickly learn that time management is one of the most important skills you can master. Your shift can go from calm to chaos in a matter of seconds, and it's easy to feel overwhelmed when you're juggling patient care, charting, and unexpected emergencies. The truth is, you can't do it all at once—but you can learn how to prioritize, stay organized, and make the most of your time. This chapter will guide you through practical strategies to manage your workload, reduce stress, and avoid the dreaded burnout that can creep up if you're not careful.

Prioritizing Tasks: Understanding What's Urgent vs. Important

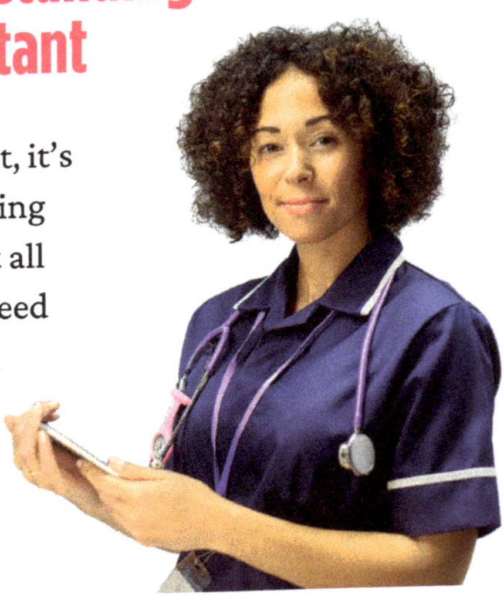

When you're staring at a long to-do list, it's tempting to just dive in and start tackling tasks as they come. But in nursing, not all tasks are created equal. Some things need immediate attention, while others can wait a bit longer. The key to staying on top of your workload is learning how to differentiate between what's urgent and what's important.

- **Urgent tasks** are those that demand immediate action. For example, if a patient's oxygen saturation drops suddenly, that's a task that can't wait.
- **Important tasks**, on the other hand, may not need your immediate attention but are still critical to overall patient care—like updating a care plan or completing a detailed chart.

One way to keep track of priorities is to use the "ABCDE" method, which focuses on patient safety:

- **A**: Airway issues come first.
- **B**: Breathing problems are next.
- **C**: Circulation (like sudden drops in blood pressure).
- **D**: Disability or neurological changes.
- **E**: Exposure (assessing for injuries or other unseen conditions).

As you get more experience, **prioritizing** will become second nature. **Until then**, don't hesitate to ask for **guidance** from your preceptor or colleagues when you're unsure what to tackle first.

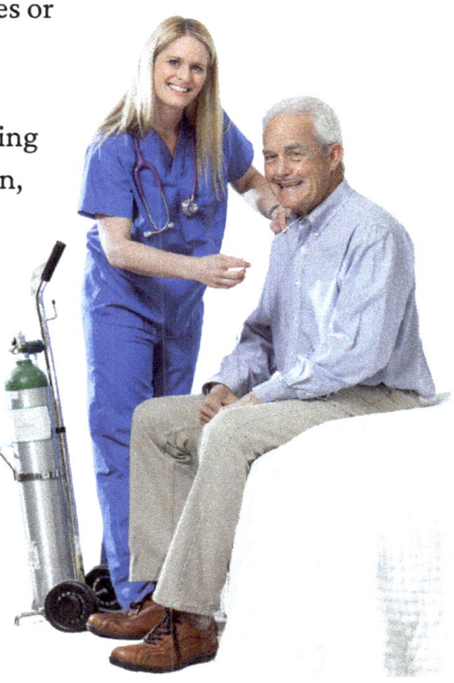

Creating a Daily Routine to Maximize Productivity

Even in the busiest environments, establishing a routine can help you stay focused and efficient. While every shift is different, you can create a flexible framework to guide your day:

- **Start Strong with Report**

Begin your shift by getting a thorough handoff report. Take notes, ask questions, and identify any immediate tasks or potential issues for each patient. This is your roadmap for the day.

- **Plan Your Priorities**

After report, take a few minutes to map out your day. Look at your patients' schedules for medications, treatments, and tests. Build your timeline around those, but leave room for flexibility—because something will come up.

- **Cluster Your Care**

Instead of running back and forth between patient rooms, try to group tasks together. For example, when you're in a patient's room to check vital signs, use that time to assess their condition, reposition them if needed, and ensure they have everything they need.

- **Stay on Top of Charting**

Documentation can easily pile up if you don't stay on top of it. Aim to chart as you go, even if it's just brief notes that you expand on later. This prevents the dreaded end-of-shift scramble.

- **Check In Regularly**

Take a few minutes every couple of hours to review your plan and adjust as needed. A quick reset can keep you on track and help you stay proactive instead of reactive.

Avoiding Burnout: Recognizing the Signs and Taking Action

Burnout is a very real challenge in nursing, especially for new grads. The long hours, emotional demands, and constant pressure to keep up can take a toll on even the most passionate nurses. But recognizing the early signs of burnout and taking steps to protect your well-being can make all the difference.

Signs of Burnout:

- Constant fatigue, even after a full night's sleep
- Feeling emotionally drained or detached from your work
- A sense of dread before your shifts
- Difficulty concentrating or making decisions
- Frequent headaches, stomach issues, or other physical symptoms

If you notice these signs, it's time to take action.

Strategies to Prevent and Manage Burnout:

- **Set Boundaries**

It's easy to say "yes" to every extra shift or task when you're new and eager to impress, but overcommitting can lead to exhaustion. Learn to set healthy boundaries and say "no" when needed.

- **Take Breaks**

Yes, you're busy—but you're also human. Even a 5-minute break to step outside, drink some water, or practice deep breathing can help reset your mind and body.

- **Find an Outlet**

Nursing can be emotionally intense. Whether it's journaling, talking to a trusted colleague, or seeking professional support, find a way to process your feelings and decompress.

- **Prioritize Self-Care**

Outside of work, focus on the basics: sleep, nutrition, exercise, and spending time with loved ones. The better you take care of yourself, the better you'll be able to care for your patients.

- **Lean on Your Team**

Remember, you're not alone. Your colleagues understand the challenges you're facing, and many of them have been in your shoes. Don't hesitate to ask for help or share your struggles—it's a sign of strength, not weakness.

Time management is a skill that takes time to develop, but by prioritizing tasks, creating a daily routine, and protecting your mental health, you'll set yourself up for success. Remember, nursing is a team effort, and you don't have to figure it all out on your own. With practice, patience, and a little grace for yourself, you'll find your rhythm—and thrive in your new role.

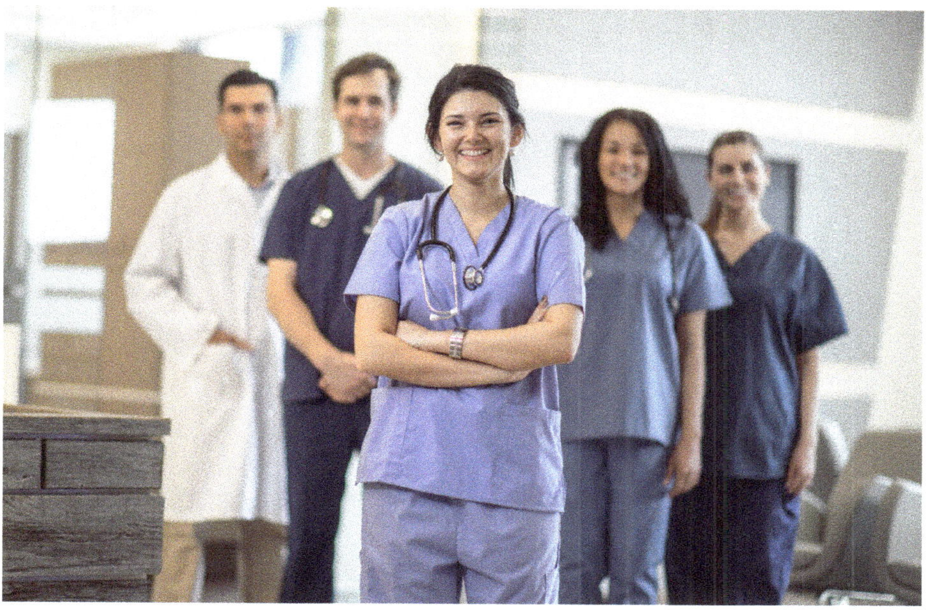

Chapter **Three**

THE IMPORTANCE OF Communication

If there's one skill that will make or break your nursing career, it's communication. Whether you're explaining a treatment plan to a worried patient, collaborating with a colleague during a hectic shift, or receiving feedback from a supervisor, the way you communicate can shape the outcomes of every interaction. Nurses are often the bridge between patients, families, and the rest of the healthcare team, which means your ability to listen, clarify, and share information effectively is critical. The good news? Communication is a skill you can build and refine with practice.

In this chapter, we'll explore how to navigate three essential areas of communication: talking with patients and families, collaborating with your healthcare team, and learning to give and receive feedback constructively.

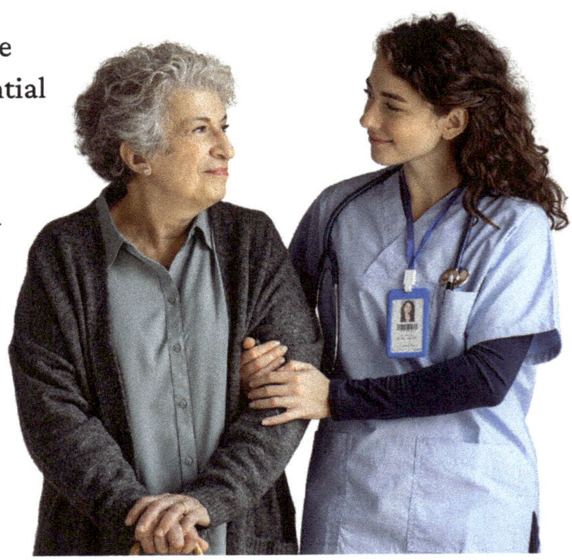

Communicating Effectively with Patients and Their Families

Let's start with one of your most important roles: being the voice of calm, compassion, and clarity for your patients and their loved ones. For many people, being in a hospital or healthcare setting is stressful and scary. They're looking to you not only for answers but also for reassurance.

Here are a few tips to make your patient and family interactions smoother:

- **Be Present.** When you're speaking with a patient or their family, give them your full attention. Eye contact, open body language, and active listening can go a long way in making them feel heard and valued—even if you only have a few minutes to spare.
- **Simplify Medical Jargon.** You've spent years learning complicated terms, but patients don't have the same background. Always translate complex medical language into something simple and easy to understand. For example, instead of saying "You're experiencing tachycardia," try "Your heart rate is beating faster than normal."
- **Empathy Over Answers.** You won't always have the answers, and that's okay. What patients and families often need most is empathy. A simple "I know this is hard, and we're doing everything we can to help" can bring them more comfort than an overly detailed explanation.

- **Ask Questions.** Don't assume you understand what a patient or family member is feeling—ask them. "What concerns you the most right now?" or "What questions do you have for me?" opens the door for meaningful conversations.

Collaborating with Healthcare Professionals

As a nurse, you'll be working side by side with doctors, respiratory therapists, pharmacists, techs, and many others. Each person on the healthcare team plays a vital role in patient care, and effective collaboration ensures that nothing falls through the cracks.

Here's how you can foster strong teamwork:

- **Be Respectful.** No matter the person's role, treat everyone on the team with respect. A tech or transporter can be just as critical to patient care as a surgeon, and building mutual respect will make your work environment more positive and productive.
- **Speak Up When Needed.** If you notice something that doesn't seem right—whether it's a medication order, a treatment plan, or a patient's condition—don't hesitate to voice your concerns. Remember, patient safety is everyone's responsibility.
- **Be Clear and Concise.** Healthcare is fast-paced, so when you're communicating with other professionals, keep your message focused. Use tools like SBAR (Situation, Background, Assessment, Recommendation) to

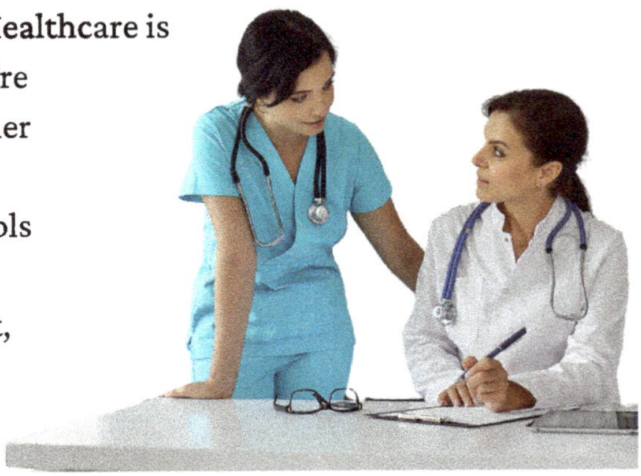

organize your thoughts and present information quickly and effectively.

- **Ask for Help.** You're new, and no one expects you to know everything. Don't be afraid to lean on your team when you're unsure about something—they've been where you are and will likely appreciate your willingness to learn.

Giving and Receiving Constructive Feedback

Feedback is a gift—it helps you grow, improve, and become the best nurse you can be. But let's be honest: it's not always easy to give or receive feedback, especially in a high-pressure environment like healthcare. Here's how to handle it like a pro:

When Giving Feedback:

- **Be Specific.** Instead of saying, "You're not doing this right," focus on specific behaviors or actions: "I noticed that during your dressing change, you forgot to check for redness around the wound. It's important to assess the area to monitor for infection."
- **Be Kind.** Feedback doesn't have to be harsh to be effective. Frame your suggestions as opportunities for improvement, not criticisms.
- **Offer Solutions.** Don't just point out what went wrong—help your colleague find a way to do it better next time.

When Receiving Feedback:

- **Listen Without Defensiveness.** It's natural to feel a little hurt or embarrassed when someone points out a mistake, but try to separate the feedback from your emotions. They're not criticizing you as a person—they're helping you grow as a professional.

- **Ask Questions.** If the feedback isn't clear, ask for clarification. "Can you show me how you would approach that differently?" is a great way to learn from constructive criticism.
- **Thank the Person.** Even if the feedback stings, thank the person for taking the time to help you improve. It shows maturity and professionalism.

Putting It All Together

Great communication takes practice, patience, and humility. You'll make mistakes along the way—we all do—but every conversation is an opportunity to learn and grow. Remember, you're not just communicating to get a task done; you're building relationships, ensuring patient safety, and fostering a collaborative environment.

When you prioritize clear, compassionate communication, you'll not only become a more effective nurse—you'll also make a lasting impact on your patients, their families, and your team.

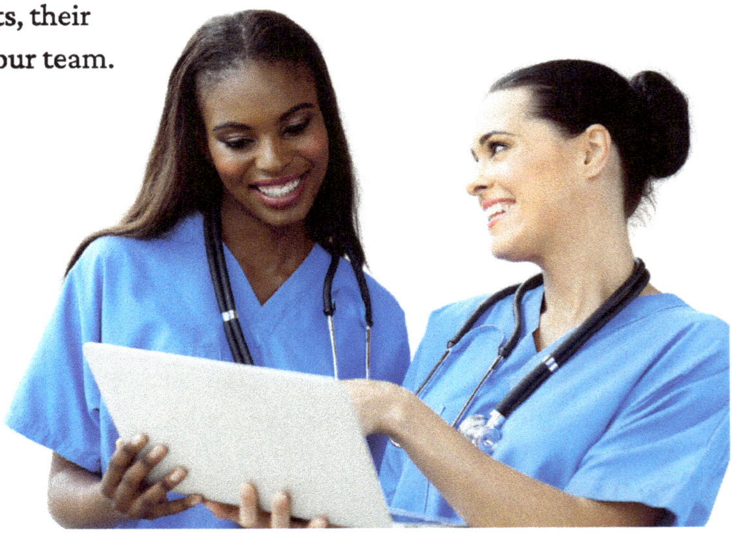

Chapter **Four**

THE BASICS OF Patient Safety

Patient safety is at the heart of everything you do as a nurse. It's not just a checklist to follow—it's a mindset, a responsibility, and a commitment to ensuring that every patient receives the best care possible in a safe environment. Whether it's preventing infections, properly administering medications, or simply double-checking a chart, your actions have a direct impact on your patients' well-being.

As a new nurse, it's easy to get caught up in the whirlwind of tasks, but never forget that patient safety always comes first. In this chapter, we'll go over the essentials of patient safety, from understanding protocols to using PPE correctly.

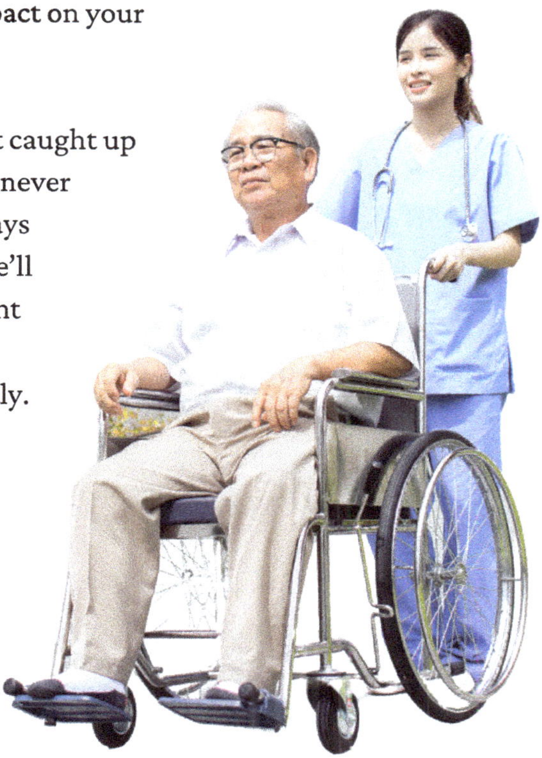

Understanding Patient Safety Protocols

Let's start with the basics: patient safety protocols. These are the guidelines and procedures that help prevent errors, injuries, and complications. They may vary slightly between facilities, but the core principles are universal. Following them isn't just about compliance—it's about creating a culture of safety for your patients and your team.

Take time to familiarize yourself with your facility's specific safety protocols as soon as you start working. These could include procedures for medication administration, fall prevention strategies, or the correct way to transfer patients. If you're unsure about something, ask. Nobody expects you to know everything from day one, but they will expect you to follow safety measures consistently.

Here's a tip: Always use critical thinking. Protocols are your guide, but your judgment matters too. For example, if a patient's condition changes, don't hesitate to reassess what's safest for them—even if it means deviating slightly from a routine practice.

The Importance of Infection Control

Infection control is one of the most vital components of patient safety. Hospital-acquired infections (HAIs) are a serious problem in healthcare, and as a nurse, you're on the front lines of preventing them.

It all starts with the basics: **hand hygiene.** You've probably heard this a thousand times during nursing school, but washing your hands before and after every patient interaction truly cannot be overstated. Use the "20-second rule" with soap and water, or an alcohol-based hand sanitizer if your hands aren't visibly dirty.

Beyond hand hygiene, you'll need to be vigilant about preventing the spread of infections through proper cleaning of equipment, isolation precautions, and maintaining a sterile field during procedures. Always follow your facility's infection control policies, and don't cut corners.

One of the best habits you can develop early on is to think ahead. For example, if you know you're about to perform a wound dressing change, gather all the supplies you'll need in advance so you're not repeatedly going in and out of the room, potentially contaminating the environment.

Proper Use of Personal Protective Equipment (PPE)

By now, you're no stranger to personal protective equipment (PPE). Masks, gloves, gowns, and face shields aren't just for your safety—they're also critical for protecting your patients.

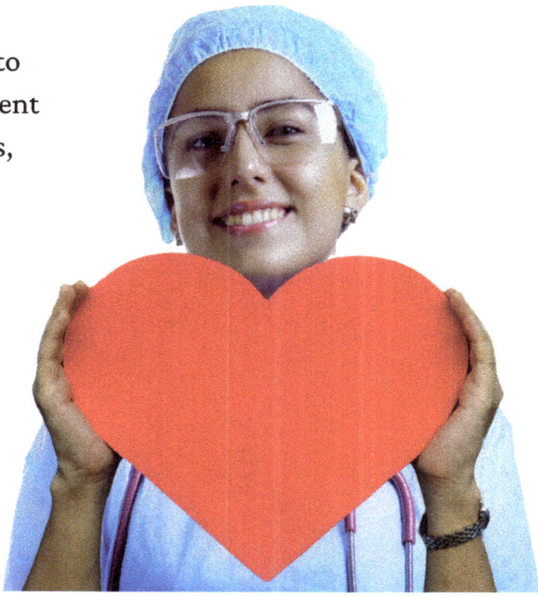

The key to PPE is using it correctly every single time. Here are a few reminders:

- **Know what PPE is required for each situation.** Whether it's standard precautions for general patient care or droplet precautions for a patient with a respiratory infection, you need to understand what's appropriate.
- **Follow proper donning and doffing techniques.** Believe it or not, many infections are spread because healthcare workers remove their PPE improperly. Learn the correct order (for example, gloves off first, then gown, then mask) and practice it until it's second nature.
- **Don't reuse disposable PPE.** While some facilities may have protocols for reusing certain items during shortages, always follow your employer's guidelines.
- **Speak up if supplies are low.** If you notice a shortage of gloves, masks, or gowns, report it immediately. Patient safety—and your own safety—depends on having the right equipment available.

Remember, PPE is your armor. It might feel tedious at times to suit up for every patient interaction, but it's a small inconvenience compared to the risk of spreading infection.

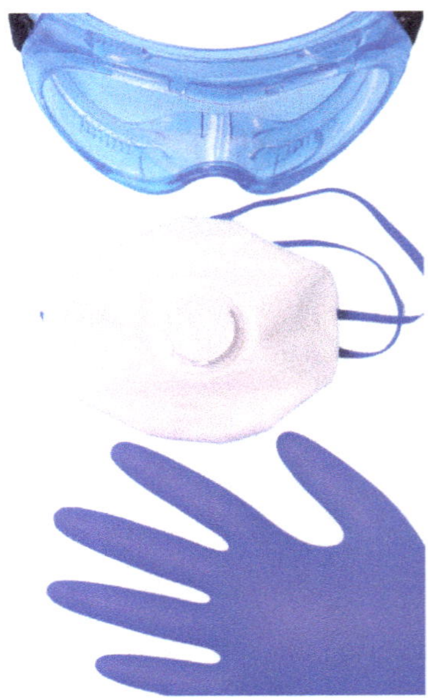

Final Thoughts

Patient safety is the foundation of quality care, and as a new nurse, you have the power to make a real difference. By understanding and adhering to safety protocols, prioritizing infection control, and using PPE correctly, you'll be protecting not only your patients but also yourself and your team.

Think of patient safety as a habit, not just a task. The more mindful you are about these basics, the more confident you'll feel in providing excellent care—and the more trust you'll earn from your patients and colleagues. After all, a safe patient is a happy patient. And at the end of the day, that's what nursing is all about.

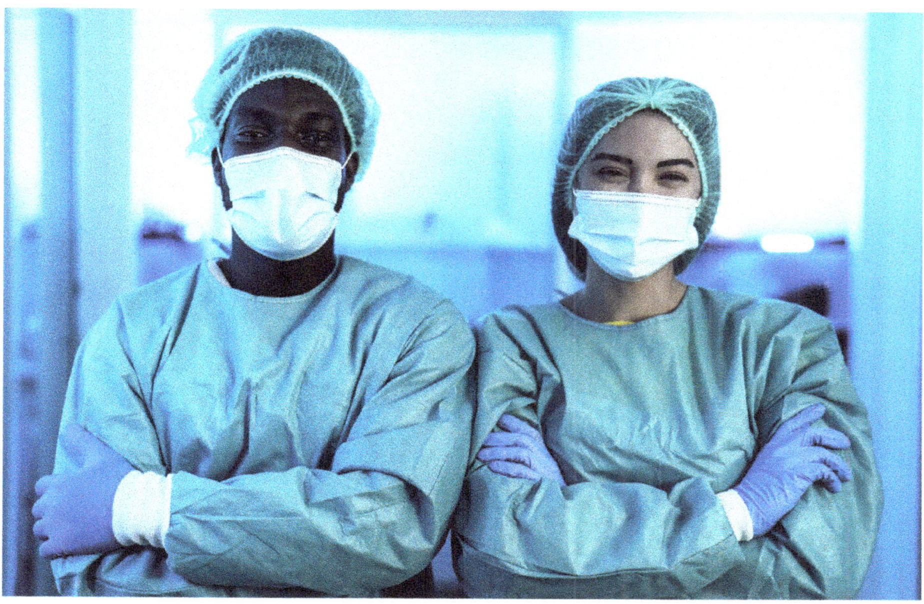

Chapter **Five**

DOCUMENTATION & Legal Awareness

As a nurse, documentation is one of the most important—and sometimes overlooked—parts of your job. It might not feel as rewarding as providing hands-on care or as urgent as responding to a critical situation, but proper documentation is the backbone of safe, effective, and legal nursing practice. There's a saying in healthcare: "If it's not documented, it didn't happen." And let me tell you, those words will become your mantra.

Your charting is not just a record of what you've done; it's a legal document, a communication tool, and a way to ensure continuity of care for your patients. In this chapter, we'll dive into the essentials of documentation, explore your legal responsibilities as a nurse, and talk about how to protect yourself in an increasingly litigious world.

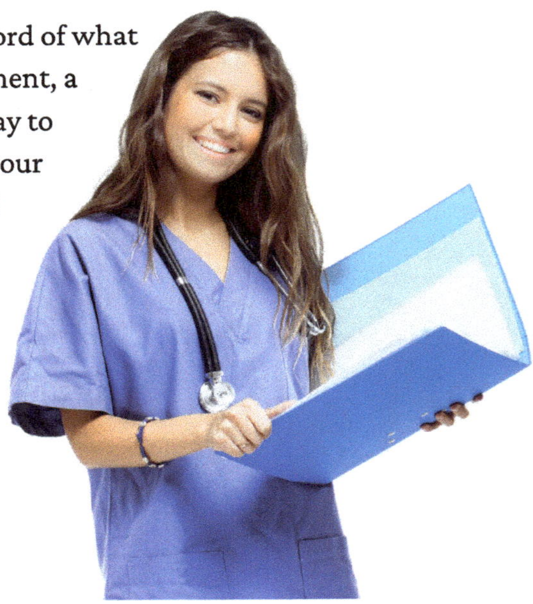

The Golden Rule: If It's Not Documented, It Didn't Happen

Let's start with this: Documentation is your best friend. Whether you've administered medication, educated a patient, or noticed a change in their condition, it needs to be recorded clearly, accurately, and promptly. Why? Because documentation serves many purposes:

- **Communication:** Your notes help other healthcare providers understand what's been done, what's needed, and any changes in the patient's condition. Without proper documentation, critical information can fall through the cracks.
- **Legal protection:** If a situation arises where your actions are questioned—whether it's a medication error or a patient complaint—your documentation is your evidence. It shows what you did, when you did it, and why.
- **Quality care:** Accurate charting ensures the next nurse, doctor, or therapist knows exactly what's happening with the patient. It's all about continuity of care.

Pro tips for effective documentation:

- **Be specific and objective**: Write what you see, hear, or do without adding assumptions or opinions. Instead of saying, "Patient seemed upset," write, "Patient stated, 'I feel worried about my surgery tomorrow.'"
- **Document in real-time**: Waiting too long to chart can lead to forgetting details or making errors. Chart as soon as possible after providing care.

- **Use approved abbreviations:** Stick to facility-approved abbreviations to avoid confusion or misinterpretation.

Understanding HIPAA and Patient Confidentiality

Patient confidentiality is not just a legal requirement—it's an ethical obligation. The Health Insurance Portability and Accountability Act (HIPAA) sets strict standards for how patient information is handled, shared, and stored. Violating HIPAA, even unintentionally, can result in serious consequences for you, your employer, and the patient.

Here are the basics of protecting patient confidentiality:

- **Share information only on a need-to-know basis:** If someone isn't directly involved in the patient's care, they don't need to know the details. This includes coworkers, friends, and family members.
- **Be mindful of your surroundings:** Avoid discussing patients in public areas like elevators, cafeterias, or hallways. Even casual comments can be overheard and lead to breaches.
- **Secure patient records:** Whether it's electronic or paper, ensure patient records are stored safely. Log out of computers, avoid sharing passwords, and keep paper charts in designated areas.

Remember, protecting patient information isn't just about avoiding legal trouble—it's about building trust. Patients need to feel confident that their personal information is safe with you.

Protecting Yourself Legally as a Nurse

Nursing is a profession with tremendous responsibility, and with that responsibility comes potential legal risks. While it's not something you want to dwell on, it's important to know how to protect yourself.

- **Follow policies and procedures:** Every facility has its own policies and protocols. Familiarize yourself with them and stick to them. If you're ever asked to do something that doesn't align with those policies, speak up or seek clarification.
- **Know your scope of practice:** Each state has a nurse practice act that outlines what you're legally allowed to do. Never perform a task you're not trained or authorized to do, even if someone asks you to.
- **Communicate concerns:** If you notice unsafe practices or feel uncomfortable with a situation, don't hesitate to escalate it. Document your concerns and report them to the appropriate supervisor.
- **Carry liability insurance:** While most employers provide some form of liability coverage, it's a good idea to have your own insurance. It offers additional protection in case you're named in a lawsuit.

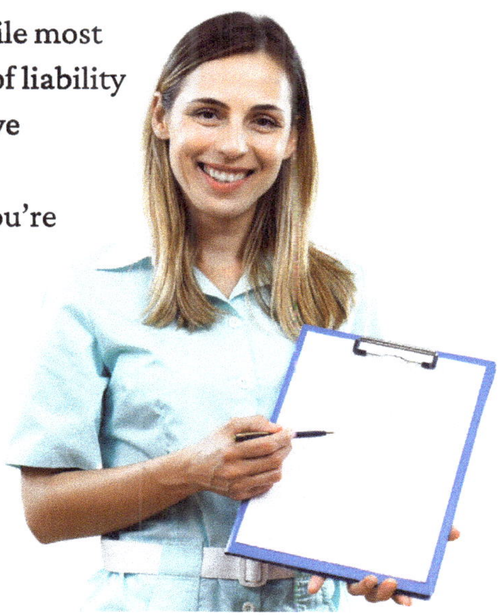

Finally, remember that your documentation is your first line of defense. If something goes wrong, the chart is the first place anyone will look. By documenting thoroughly and accurately, you're protecting not just your patients, but yourself as well.

Key Takeaways

- Always document care as if you're explaining it to a jury.
- HIPAA isn't just a set of rules—it's a cornerstone of trust in healthcare.
- Protect yourself legally by following policies, knowing your scope, and documenting everything.

Patient safety and confidentiality go hand in hand with your own legal safety. When you combine strong documentation habits with an awareness of your legal responsibilities, you're not only safeguarding your patients—you're setting yourself up for a long and successful nursing career.

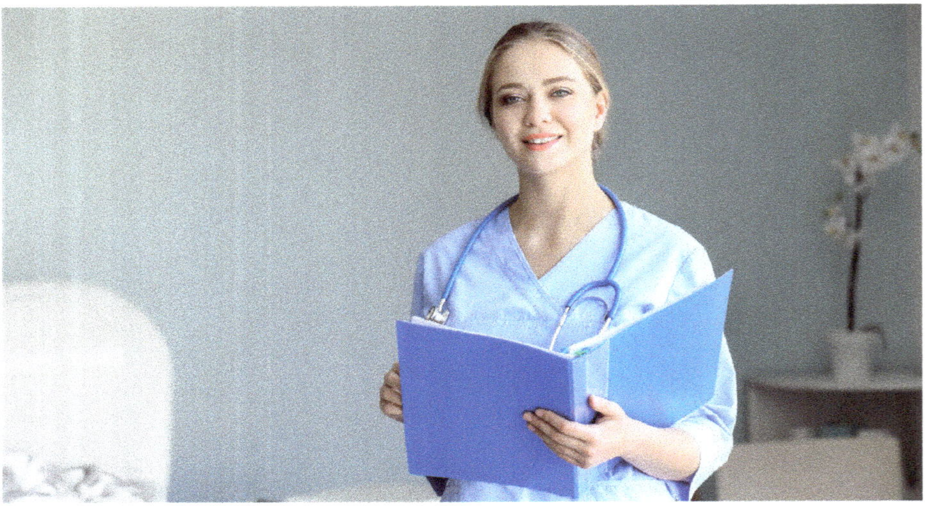

Chapter **Six**

MISTAKES IN Patient Care

No one starts their nursing career intending to make mistakes, but the truth is, mistakes can and do happen—especially when you're still finding your footing in this fast-paced and high-stakes profession. The key is to recognize the most common pitfalls, understand why they happen, and actively work to prevent them. This chapter is all about helping you navigate the tricky waters of patient care by highlighting some of the most frequent mistakes new nurses make—and, more importantly, how to avoid them.

Let's dive into these potential pitfalls and explore how simple, mindful practices can keep your patients safe and your mind at ease.

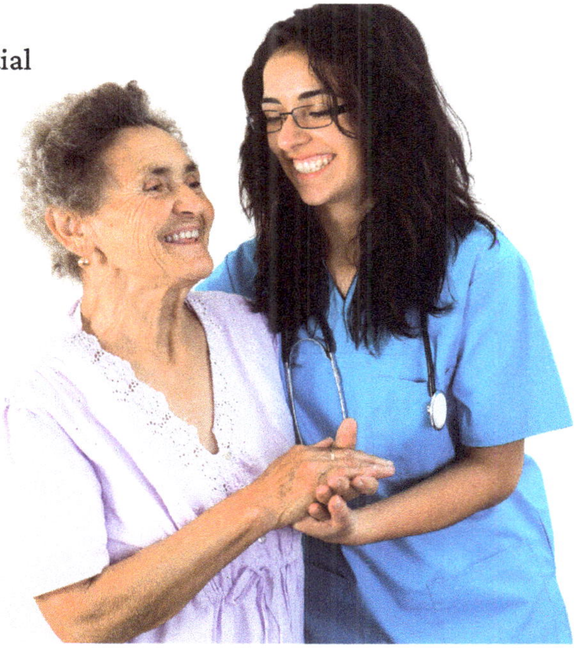

Not Asking Questions When Unsure About Something

It can feel intimidating to ask questions, especially when you're surrounded by seasoned healthcare professionals. You might worry about looking inexperienced or feel like you should already know the answer. But let me tell you this: asking questions is a strength, not a weakness.

Healthcare is complex, and you're not expected to know everything. If you're unsure about a procedure, medication, or protocol, speak up. It's better to ask for clarification than to take a guess and risk harming your patient. Most experienced nurses will appreciate your willingness to learn and would much rather answer your questions than fix a preventable mistake.

Here's a tip: Start with something like, "I just want to confirm I'm doing this correctly." This shows you're taking initiative while also prioritizing safety.

Failing to Double-Check Medications Before Administration

Medications save lives—but they can also cause harm if administered incorrectly. One of the most dangerous mistakes a nurse can make is failing to double-check medications before giving them to a patient.

To avoid this, always follow the "Five Rights" of medication administration:

- **Right patient** – Make sure you're giving the medication to the correct patient by checking their wristband and asking for their name and date of birth.
- **Right medication** – Double-check the prescription and make sure it matches the label on the medication.
- **Right dose** – Verify that the dosage is correct, especially when measuring liquids or splitting tablets.
- **Right time** – Administer the medication at the right time to maintain its effectiveness.
- **Right route** – Confirm whether the medication should be given orally, intravenously, or another route.

If you're ever in doubt, take a moment to verify the order with the prescribing provider or pharmacist. A quick pause could prevent a major error.

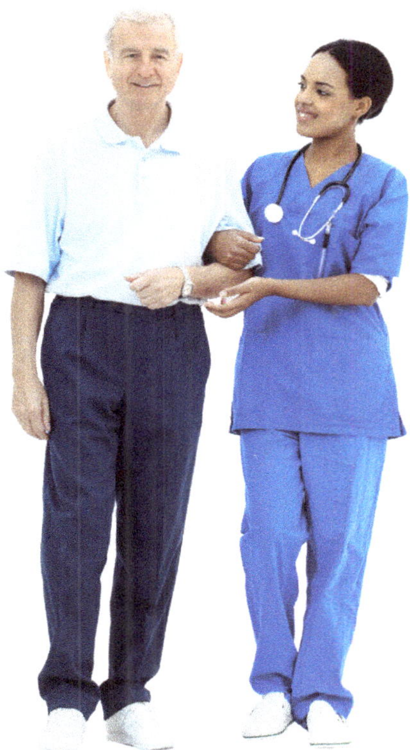

Neglecting to Wash Hands Before and After Patient Contact

It sounds almost too simple, doesn't it? But hand hygiene is one of the most effective ways to prevent infections and keep both you and your patients safe.

When you're rushing from one task to another, it's easy to overlook this step. But remember: every patient deserves clean hands. Wash your hands before and after touching a patient, even if you're wearing gloves. This isn't just about meeting infection control standards; it's about showing your patients that their safety matters to you.

Here's a pro tip: If your hands are getting dry from frequent washing, invest in a high-quality hand lotion that's compatible with hospital-grade sanitizers.

Ignoring Changes in a Patient's Condition

Patients often give subtle clues when something is wrong. It's your job to notice those changes and act on them quickly.

Maybe a patient's heart rate is climbing, their breathing is labored, or their mental status seems off. These could be early warning signs of deterioration, and ignoring them could lead to serious consequences. Trust your instincts—if something doesn't seem right, it probably isn't.

One strategy is to use the SBAR technique (Situation, Background, Assessment, Recommendation) when communicating concerns to a provider. It's a clear, concise way to ensure your observations are taken seriously.

Not Verifying Patient Identity Before Providing Care

Picture this: You walk into a patient's room, see their medication tray, and administer the meds without confirming their identity. Moments later, you realize you've given the wrong patient the wrong medication. It's a nightmare scenario, but it happens more often than you'd think.

To avoid this, always verify your patient's identity using two identifiers—usually their name and date of birth—before administering medications, performing procedures, or providing any care. Even if you think you know the patient well, don't skip this step. A small pause for verification can prevent a huge error.

Improper Handling of Medical Equipment

From IV pumps to ventilators, nurses interact with a wide range of medical equipment every day. While these tools are designed to save lives, improper use can cause harm.

Take the time to familiarize yourself with the equipment you'll be using. Many hospitals offer in-services or training sessions—don't hesitate to attend them, even if you think you already know the basics. If you're unsure how to operate a device, ask for help or consult the manual. Remember, it's better to pause and ensure you're using the equipment correctly than to risk injuring a patient.

Final Thoughts

Mistakes in patient care are often the result of rushing, assumptions, or hesitation to ask for help. By slowing down, following protocols, and staying vigilant, you can prevent many of these errors. Every nurse, no matter how experienced, has made mistakes—but what sets great nurses apart is their commitment to learning from those mistakes and improving every day.

Patient care is a team effort, and when you focus on communication, attention to detail, and continuous learning, you'll not only avoid these common pitfalls but also build a reputation as a safe and competent nurse. Keep striving for excellence—it's what your patients deserve.

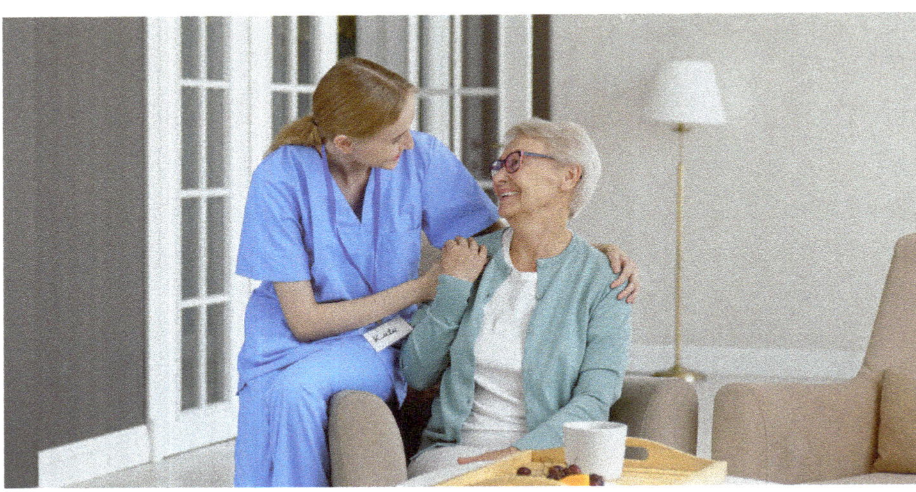

Chapter **Seven**

MISTAKES IN Communication

Communication is the cornerstone of effective nursing care. It's how we ensure continuity of care, build trust with patients and families, and collaborate with our colleagues. But even with the best intentions, communication can sometimes go awry. Whether it's a misunderstood order or a missed piece of critical information during a shift handoff, these lapses can have serious consequences. The good news is that with some awareness and practice, you can avoid these common communication mistakes and become a more effective, compassionate, and reliable communicator.

Not Effectively Communicating During Handoffs or Shift Reports

One of the most crucial moments in a nurse's shift is the handoff. This is when you pass the baton to the next nurse, sharing vital information about your patients. It's easy to rush through this process, especially at the end of a long shift, but doing so can leave critical details unshared.

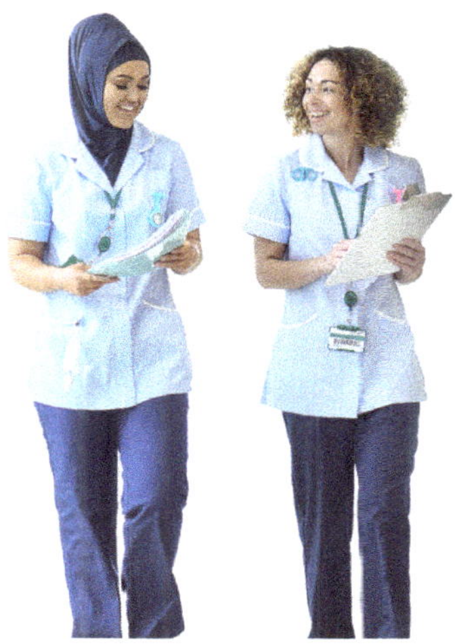

Ensuring Critical Information is Passed On: Make a checklist or use a standardized handoff protocol like SBAR (Situation, Background, Assessment, Recommendation). This ensures you don't miss any important details, such as changes in condition, pending tests, or specific patient needs. Clear, concise, and thorough communication can prevent misunderstandings and errors in care.

Failing to Clarify Unclear Orders from a Physician

Doctors are busy, and sometimes their orders can be unclear or seem incomplete. It's your job to make sure you fully understand what's being asked of you.

Why It's Okay to Seek Clarification: Asking questions doesn't make you look incompetent; it shows you care about doing the right thing. Whether it's a medication dosage that seems off or a treatment plan that doesn't quite make sense, always seek clarification. Use tools like read-back techniques to confirm that you've understood the orders correctly.

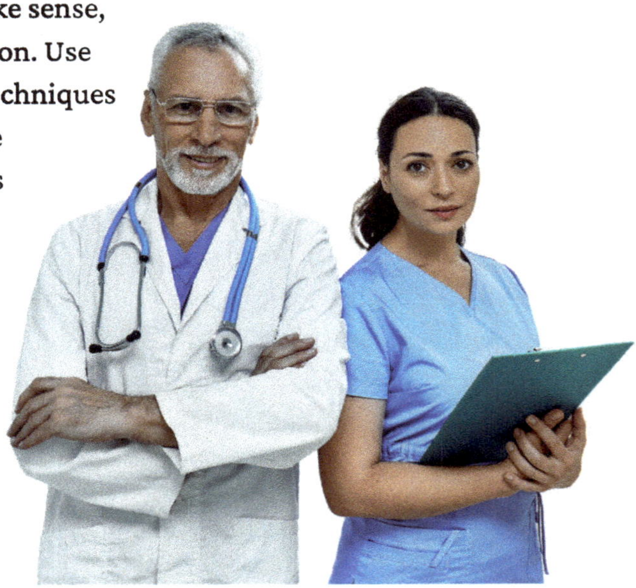

Using Medical Jargon with Patients and Families

Medical jargon is second nature to healthcare professionals, but for patients and their families, it can be confusing and intimidating.

Adapting Your Language for Better Understanding: Use plain language whenever possible. Instead of saying "myocardial infarction," say "heart attack." Instead of "hypertension," say "high blood pressure." Remember, the goal is to make sure your patients and their families fully understand their conditions and treatments. This builds trust and helps them feel more involved in their care.

Avoiding Difficult Conversations with Patients or Families

No one likes delivering bad news, but avoiding difficult conversations can leave patients and families in the dark and feeling unsupported.

Navigating End-of-Life Care or Difficult Diagnoses: Approach these conversations with empathy and honesty. Use open-ended questions to understand their concerns and feelings. Offer clear, straightforward information, and provide emotional support. Sometimes, just listening can make a huge difference. You don't need to have all the answers, but you do need to be present and compassionate.

Not Addressing Conflict Within the Healthcare Team

Conflict is inevitable in any workplace, but in a healthcare setting, unresolved issues can impact patient care.

The Importance of Resolving Misunderstandings: Address conflicts directly and professionally. Use "I" statements to express your feelings without blaming others (e.g., "I feel concerned when..."). Seek to understand the other person's perspective and find a resolution that works for both parties. Remember, a harmonious team is essential for providing the best patient care.

By being mindful of these common communication mistakes and actively working to improve your skills, you'll not only become a more effective nurse but also a trusted and valued member of your healthcare team. Communication is key, and mastering it is one of the best things you can do for your career and your patients.

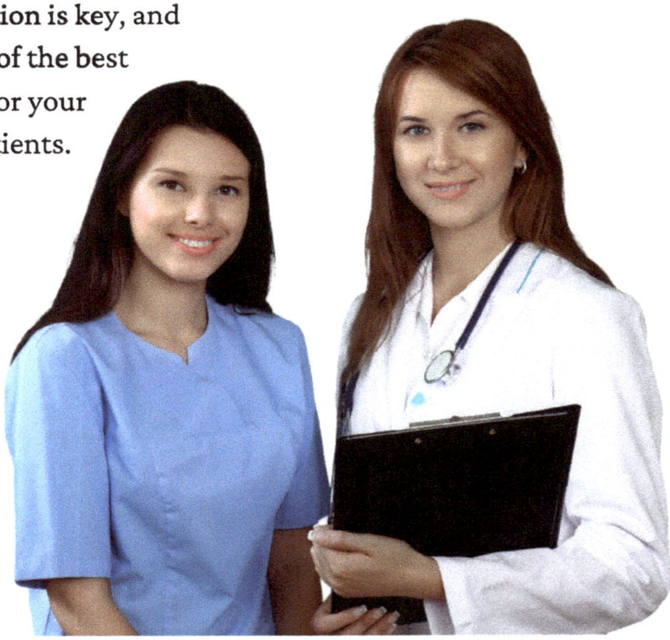

Chapter **Eight**

ERRORS IN Documentation

Let's be honest—documentation might not be your favorite part of nursing, but it's one of the most important. It's not just about "checking the box" to say you've done your job; it's about creating a clear, accurate record of the care you provide. Documentation is how you communicate with the rest of the healthcare team, protect yourself legally, and, most importantly, ensure that your patients receive safe and consistent care.

That said, mistakes in documentation are common, especially for new nurses who are juggling a steep learning curve and a fast-paced environment. In this chapter, we'll explore some of the most frequent documentation errors and how you can avoid them by staying accurate, factual, and timely in your charting.

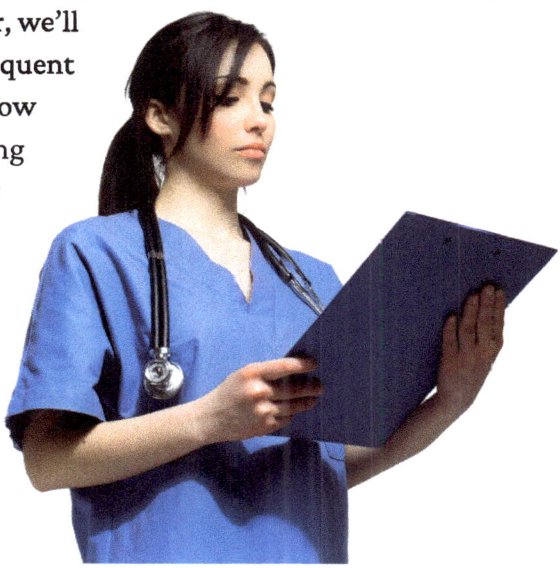

Not Properly Documenting Patient Care

"If it's not documented, it didn't happen." You've probably heard this saying a hundred times in nursing school, and for good reason—it's the golden rule of documentation. Yet, in the hustle and bustle of a busy shift, it's easy to forget to jot down something you did for a patient.

Whether it's a medication you administered, an assessment you completed, or even a conversation with a patient's family, failing to document it means there's no record of it ever happening. This can lead to confusion among the healthcare team, gaps in care, and even legal consequences if there's ever a question about what was done.

How to Avoid This Mistake:

- Make it a habit to document immediately after completing a task whenever possible. Don't rely on your memory to catch up later—you're busy, and details can slip through the cracks.
- Use tools like checklists or notes to keep track of what you've done if you can't chart right away, but make sure to transfer that information into the official record as soon as you can.

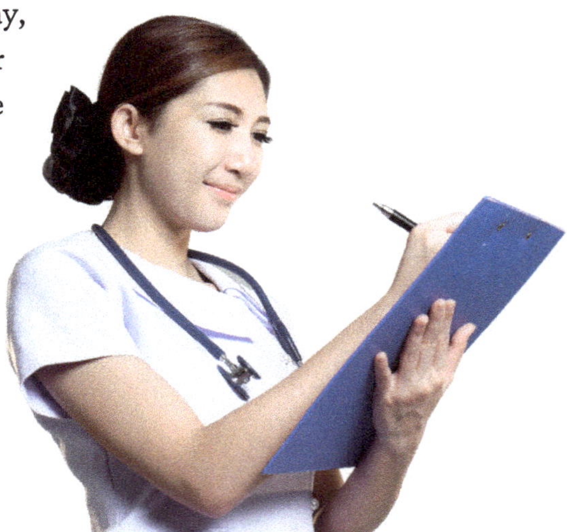

The Importance of Timely & Accurate Charting

Imagine this scenario: you check on a patient and notice their oxygen saturation has dropped significantly, but you forget to chart it until hours later—or worse, you forget altogether. Timely documentation ensures that important information is communicated to the entire team in real-time, which can literally save lives.

Accuracy is just as important. Misdocumenting a patient's vital signs, medications, or treatments can lead to incorrect decisions by other team members, creating a ripple effect of errors.

How to Avoid This Mistake:

- Develop a rhythm for documenting throughout your shift. Set mental reminders to chart after key tasks like medication administration, dressing changes, or assessments.
- Double-check your entries for accuracy before submitting them, especially when entering vital signs or medication dosages.

Charting Before Completing a Task

Pre-charting might seem like a time-saver, but it's a dangerous habit that can lead to serious consequences. If something changes with the patient—or if the task doesn't get done at all—your documentation won't match reality. This can cause confusion, miscommunication, and even put your patient at risk.

Why It's Tempting:

We've all had those moments when the to-do list is overwhelming, and pre-documenting feels like a shortcut to lighten the load. However, it's a practice that can backfire quickly.

How to Avoid This Mistake:

- Only document what you've completed. If a task remains unfinished, make a note for yourself as a reminder, but leave the charting until it's done.

Failing to Include Objective Data in Documentation

Your documentation isn't the place for assumptions or vague statements. For example, writing "patient seems fine" doesn't provide enough detail to guide the next nurse or the physician. Instead, focus on objective, measurable data.

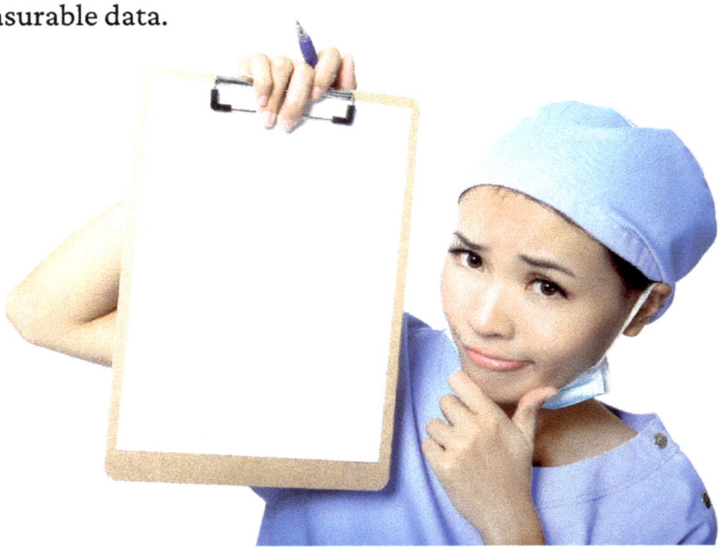

For example:

- Instead of writing "patient in pain," document, "Patient reports pain level of 8/10, localized to lower abdomen, sharp in nature."
- Instead of "wound looks better," document, "Surgical wound clean and dry, edges well-approximated, no redness, drainage, or swelling observed."

How to Avoid This Mistake:

- Use descriptive language and stick to the facts. Record what you see, hear, and measure.
- If the patient shares subjective information, include it in their words. For instance, "Patient states, 'I feel like I can't catch my breath.'"

Overlooking Discrepancies in Patient Records

It's easy to assume that what's in the chart is correct, but that's not always the case. Inaccuracies can creep in over time, especially if multiple people are updating a patient's record. If you notice something that doesn't add up—like conflicting medication lists or a vital sign that doesn't make sense—it's your responsibility to address it.

How to Avoid This Mistake:

- Cross-check patient records, especially during handoffs, to ensure consistency.
- If you notice discrepancies, don't ignore them. Clarify with the team or verify directly with the patient.

The Bottom Line

Documentation is more than just a requirement; it's a lifeline for your patients and the healthcare team. By staying timely, accurate, and factual, you not only protect yourself but also ensure that your patients receive the safest and best care possible. Remember, good documentation is a skill, and like any skill, it gets easier with practice.

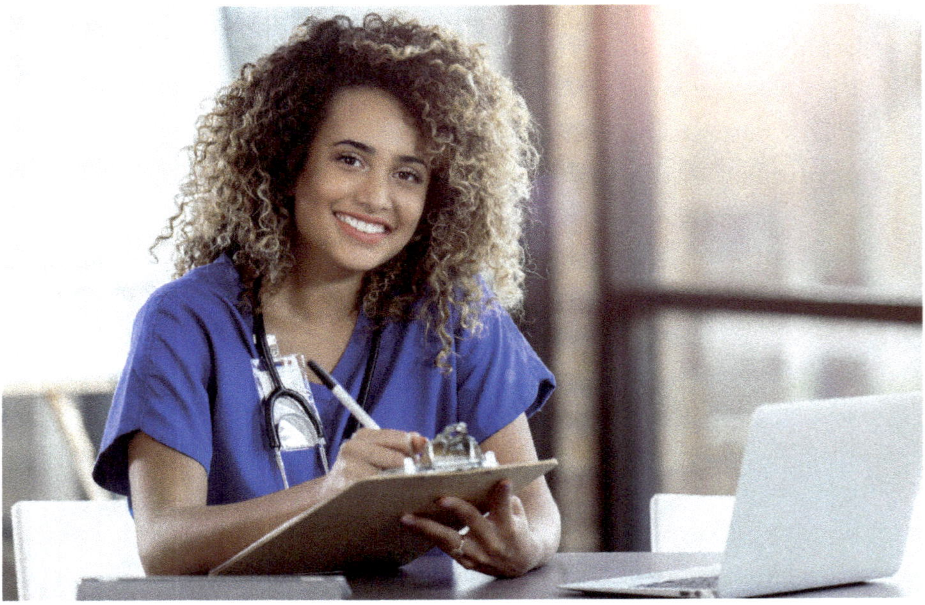

Chapter **Nine**

MISTAKES IN Prioritization

Time management is one of the biggest challenges you'll face as a new nurse. Your shift can feel like a whirlwind of patient care, documentation, calls from physicians, and unexpected emergencies. Some days, it might feel impossible to keep up with everything. But here's the thing: time management isn't about being perfect or doing it all—it's about working smarter, not harder.

This chapter is all about recognizing common time management mistakes and learning how to prioritize effectively. With a little planning, organization, and self-awareness, you can take control of your day instead of letting it control you.

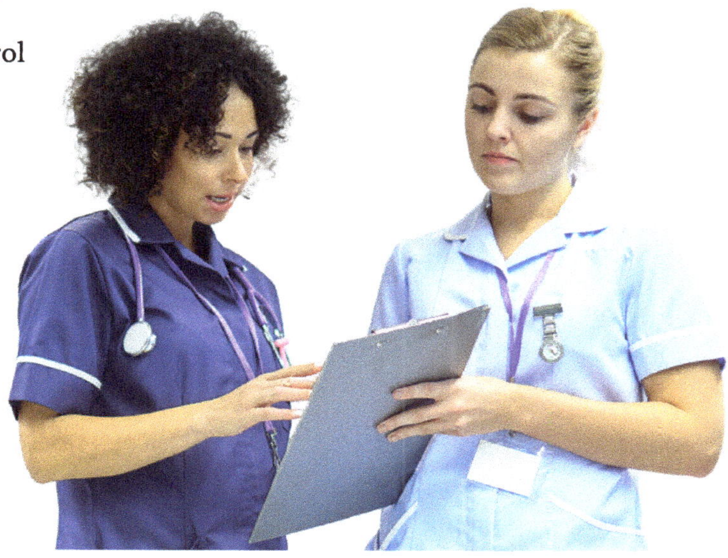

Taking on Too Much at Once

When you're new to nursing, it's tempting to say "yes" to everything. You want to prove you're capable and helpful, but taking on too much too quickly is a recipe for overwhelm and mistakes. Trying to juggle too many tasks at once can leave you feeling scattered and stressed—and that's when errors happen.

The solution? Learn to prioritize and delegate (more on that in a moment). Remember, you're part of a team. Asking for help or passing along a non-urgent task doesn't make you less competent—it makes you a more efficient and safe nurse.

Learning to Delegate Appropriately

Delegation is a skill that takes time to master. Knowing when and what to delegate can feel tricky at first, but it's a key part of managing your time. Tasks like restocking supplies, helping a patient to the bathroom, or checking vitals can often be handled by nursing assistants or other support staff.

When delegating, be clear about the task and follow up to ensure it's been completed. Communication is key—make sure the person understands the priority and has the skills to perform the task. This frees you up to focus on critical responsibilities that require your nursing expertise.

Failing to Prioritize Critical Tasks

Not all tasks are created equal. Some require immediate action, while others can wait. A common mistake for new nurses is tackling easier or less urgent tasks first, just to "get them out of the way." While this might feel satisfying, it can leave you scrambling to address more important matters later.

The key is to learn the difference between urgent and important. Start each shift by reviewing your patients' conditions and identifying critical needs. For example, administering medications on time or responding to a patient showing signs of distress should always take priority over routine tasks like changing linens.

Wasting Time Searching for Supplies

You'd be surprised how much time can slip away just looking for supplies. Running back and forth to the supply room or hunting down missing equipment eats into your already limited time.

To save yourself the frustration, get into the habit of organizing your workspace and gathering everything you need before starting a task. Whether it's wound care supplies, syringes, or medications, having everything on hand will keep you efficient and focused.

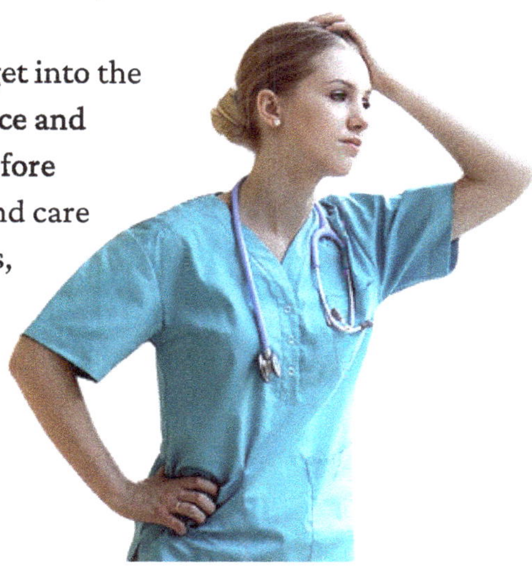

Organizing Your Workspace Efficiently

A cluttered workspace can slow you down and add unnecessary stress. At the start of your shift, take a few minutes to familiarize yourself with your unit's layout. Know where essential items are stored, and make sure your personal workspace (like your med cart or workstation) is tidy and stocked.

Keeping things organized not only saves time but also reduces errors. For example, labeling medications or keeping commonly used items in a specific spot can prevent mistakes and speed up your workflow.

Not Preparing for Your Shift in Advance

Walking into a shift without a plan is like walking into a storm without an umbrella—you're going to feel overwhelmed quickly. One of the best habits you can develop as a nurse is preparing for your shift in advance.

Start by reviewing patient charts as soon as possible. Note important details like recent lab results, medication schedules, and care plans. Use this information to create a mental or written to-do list. Having a clear plan will help you prioritize tasks and stay focused throughout your shift.

Reviewing Patient Charts and Creating a Plan

Taking a few extra minutes to thoroughly review your patient charts can make all the difference in how smoothly your shift runs. Pay attention to:

- Scheduled medications and treatments
- Any changes in orders or care plans
- Notes from previous shifts highlighting concerns or progress

From there, map out your plan. Which patients need immediate attention? Who has procedures or labs scheduled? Which tasks can wait until later? A good plan will keep you on track, even when unexpected situations arise.

Putting It All Together

Time management is a skill that takes practice, and you're not going to get it perfect right away—and that's okay! The key is to stay flexible, learn from your mistakes, and find strategies that work for you. Over time, you'll get better at prioritizing, organizing, and planning your day so you can provide the best care possible without feeling overwhelmed.

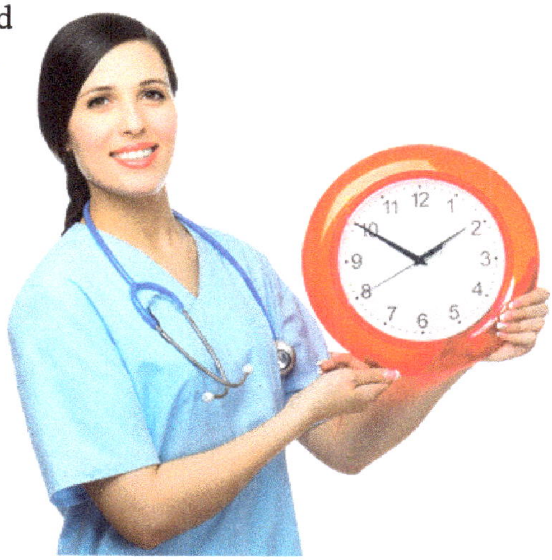

Chapter Ten

MIS-SETPS IN Ethics

As a nurse, you're not only responsible for delivering exceptional patient care but also for upholding the highest ethical and legal standards. Nursing is a profession built on trust—trust from your patients, their families, and your colleagues. Any breach of that trust, even unintentionally, can lead to serious consequences for your patients, your license, and your career.

In this chapter, we'll talk about some of the most common ethical and legal missteps new nurses encounter and, most importantly, how to avoid them. While it's normal to make small mistakes as you learn and grow, understanding your responsibilities and the potential pitfalls will help you stay on...

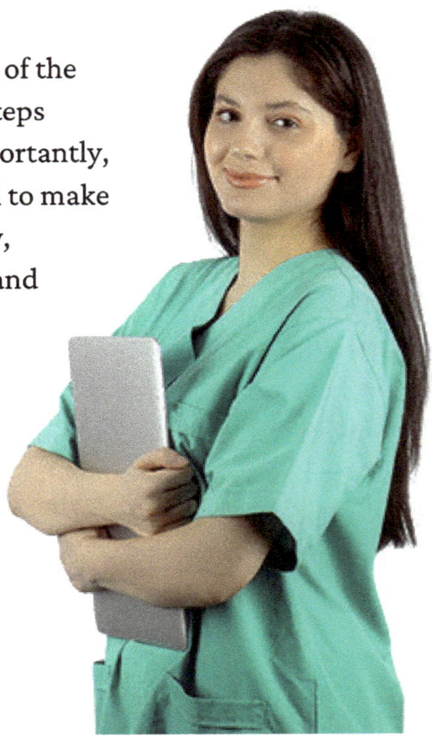

Breaching Patient Confidentiality (HIPAA Violations)

Patient confidentiality is at the core of ethical nursing practice, and it's protected by the law under the Health Insurance Portability and Accountability Act (HIPAA). While it may seem straightforward—don't share private patient information—it's surprisingly easy to unintentionally violate confidentiality in a busy workplace.

For example, discussing a patient's condition in a hallway, sharing patient updates in a crowded elevator, or even posting something vague about your day on social media can cross the line. Always ask yourself: Would this conversation or action compromise a patient's privacy?

How to Avoid HIPAA Violations:

- Discuss patient information only in private, secure settings.
- Never share patient details on social media—even anonymously.
- Double-check that you're sending faxes, emails, or lab results to the correct recipient.
- Avoid talking about patients in public spaces, even if no names are mentioned.

Protecting your patients' privacy isn't just a legal obligation; it's about respecting their dignity and trust.

Failing to Report Critical Lab Results Promptly

Imagine this: A patient's lab results come back showing dangerously high potassium levels, but you're busy finishing a medication pass. You tell yourself, "I'll follow up on that in a minute," but then you get sidetracked. Failing to act on critical lab results in a timely manner can have serious, even life-threatening, consequences.

Your role as a nurse includes recognizing the urgency of lab findings and ensuring they're communicated to the right people immediately. Delays can lead to harm for the patient and liability for you and your employer.

What You Can Do:

- Always review lab results as soon as they're available.
- Notify the physician or provider promptly if results are critical.
- Document who you contacted and what action was taken.
- If you're unsure about the significance of a lab result, don't hesitate to ask for guidance.

Remember, lab results aren't just numbers—they tell a story about your patient's condition. Acting promptly can make all the difference.

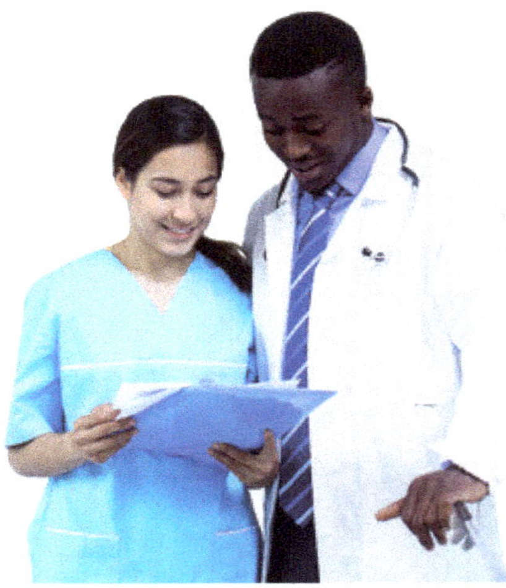

Not Documenting Incidents or Near-Misses

Mistakes happen—no one is perfect. But when an error or near-miss occurs, failing to document it can be just as problematic as the mistake itself. Incident reports aren't about pointing fingers or assigning blame; they're tools to improve patient safety and prevent future errors.

Let's say you accidentally give a patient the wrong dose of medication but catch it before harm is done. If you don't report the incident, the system flaw that allowed the error to happen might never get addressed, increasing the risk for someone else to make the same mistake.

Why Documentation Matters:

- It creates a transparent record for quality improvement.
- It protects you legally by showing you took responsibility and followed protocol.
- It ensures the healthcare team is aware of potential risks or trends.

How to Handle It:

- Always report incidents or near-misses honestly and promptly.
- Stick to the facts in your documentation—avoid subjective opinions or emotional language.
- Use incident reporting systems to improve safety protocols and reduce future risks.

Your honesty and diligence in documenting incidents can save lives and strengthen your team's processes.

Participating in Workplace Gossip

Nursing is a team effort, and the relationships you build with your colleagues can make or break your work environment. However, one of the fastest ways to erode trust and professionalism is by engaging in workplace gossip.

Whether it's talking about a colleague's mistakes, complaining about management, or discussing patients inappropriately, gossip has no place in nursing. It creates unnecessary drama, damages relationships, and can even harm patient care if it disrupts team dynamics.

How to Stay Professional:

- Focus on facts and solutions, not rumors or complaints.
- If you have concerns about a colleague's performance, address them directly or escalate them appropriately.
- Lead by example—choose not to participate in gossip, and others will notice.

Maintaining professionalism doesn't mean you can't vent or share frustrations, but do so in a constructive way and in appropriate settings. Respect for your coworkers fosters trust and creates a more positive work environment.

The Bigger Picture

Ethical and legal missteps can feel overwhelming to think about, but they're avoidable with mindfulness and a commitment to doing what's right. By protecting patient privacy, reporting critical information promptly, documenting incidents accurately, and maintaining professionalism, you'll not only keep your patients safe—you'll also build a reputation as a nurse who's trustworthy, reliable, and ethical.

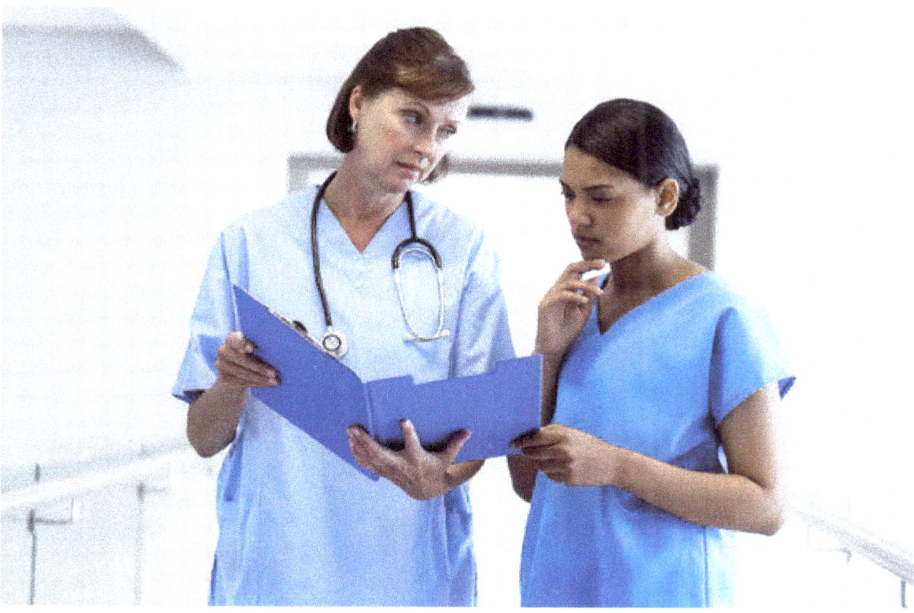

Chapter **Eleven**

MISTAKES IN TEAMWORK & Collaboration

Nursing is not a solo act—it's a team sport. While you may feel like the weight of the world is on your shoulders when caring for patients, the truth is that you're surrounded by a team of professionals all working toward the same goal: delivering safe, high-quality care. Whether you're working with other nurses, physicians, physical therapists, or dietary staff, teamwork and collaboration are the glue that holds everything together in a healthcare setting.

Unfortunately, one common mistake new nurses make is feeling like they have to handle everything alone. But here's the thing: leaning on your team, sharing responsibilities, and supporting each other doesn't just make your job easier—it also makes patient care safer and more effective. In this chapter, we'll talk about common mistakes in teamwork and how to avoid them, as well as practical ways to build strong relationships with your colleagues.

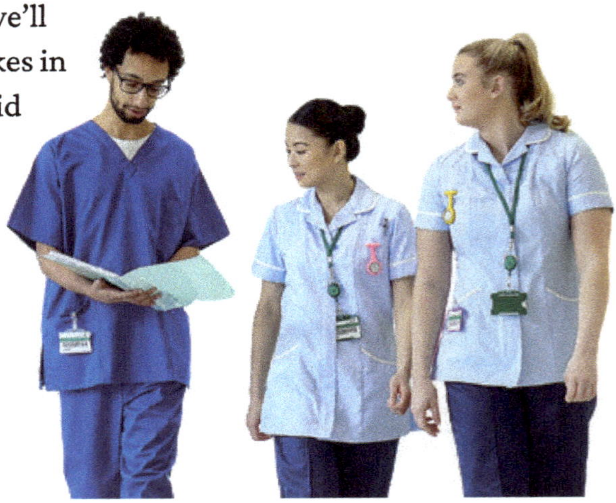

Not Seeking Help When Overwhelmed

Let's start with a reality check: You are not superhuman. There will be times when you feel like you're drowning in tasks or when you're faced with a situation you don't know how to handle. One of the biggest mistakes you can make as a new nurse is hesitating to ask for help. Whether it's because you're afraid of looking incompetent or you're trying to prove yourself, this mindset can lead to burnout—or worse, mistakes that compromise patient safety.

Why Asking for Help Is a Strength:

- It shows self-awareness and a commitment to doing what's best for the patient.
- Your team would much rather step in to support you than deal with the consequences of an avoidable error.
- Every nurse has been where you are, and most will understand that it takes time to build confidence and experience.

The key is to recognize when you're reaching your limit and to ask for help early. Whether it's asking a colleague to check a medication calculation or getting assistance with a difficult procedure, remember: teamwork is the foundation of nursing.

Failing to Support Your Colleagues

On the flip side, just as you need help sometimes, your colleagues will need support too. Nursing is emotionally and physically demanding, and small acts of kindness can make a world of difference. Ignoring a coworker who's clearly overwhelmed or dismissing their requests for help doesn't just harm your team dynamic—it can also impact patient care.

How to Build a Culture of Mutual Respect and Cooperation:

- Offer to help a colleague if you notice they're swamped, even if it's as simple as grabbing supplies or taking vital signs for their patient.
- Be approachable and nonjudgmental when someone asks for assistance.
- Remember that your teamwork sets the tone for the unit—when everyone works together, the shift goes smoother for everyone.

A team that trusts and respects each other can handle even the most chaotic days with grace.

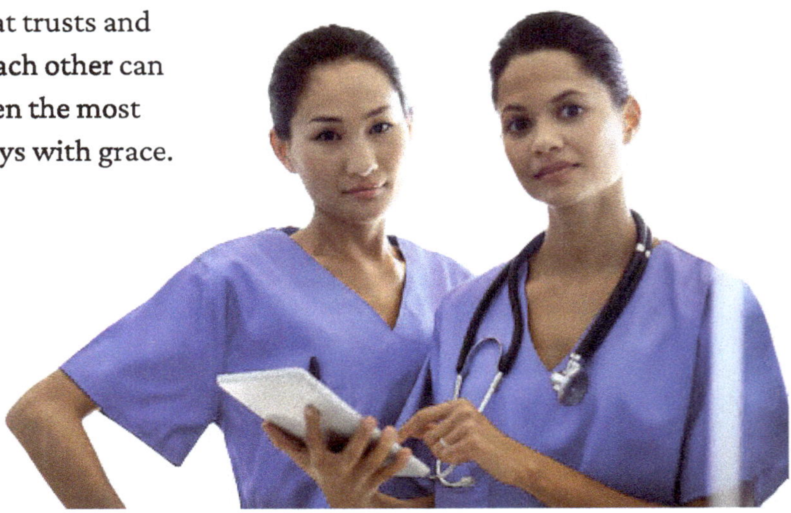

Ignoring Input from Other Healthcare Professionals

As a nurse, you're part of a larger interdisciplinary team that includes physicians, therapists, pharmacists, social workers, and more. Each of these professionals brings a unique perspective and expertise to the table, and ignoring their input can lead to missed opportunities for better patient outcomes.

For example, a physical therapist might notice something about a patient's mobility that you didn't catch, or a pharmacist might flag a potential drug interaction you weren't aware of. Valuing their input doesn't diminish your role—it enhances your ability to provide holistic care.

How to Embrace Interdisciplinary Collaboration:

- Actively listen during care team meetings or discussions.
- Don't hesitate to ask questions or seek clarification from other professionals.
- Acknowledge and respect the contributions of every member of the team, regardless of their role.

When you work collaboratively, you're not just sharing the workload—you're combining strengths to provide the best possible care for your patients.

Why Teamwork Is Essential in Nursing

The truth is, nursing can be tough. There will be days when you're exhausted, frustrated, or feeling like you're in over your head. Those are the moments when teamwork becomes your lifeline. A supportive team can lift you up, help you learn, and make even the hardest days more manageable.

And don't forget: you're not just working for your patients—you're working with them, their families, and an entire network of healthcare professionals. When you approach every interaction with a spirit of collaboration, you'll find that nursing becomes not just a job, but a deeply rewarding partnership.

In the end, the strongest nurses aren't the ones who go it alone—they're the ones who know how to lean on their team and contribute to a positive, cooperative environment. Building strong relationships with your colleagues will not only make you a better nurse, but it will also make every shift a little bit brighter.

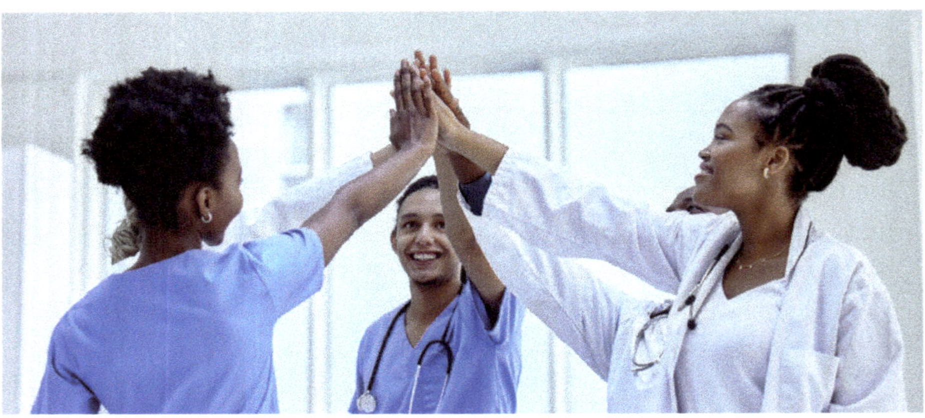

Chapter **Twelve**

PERSONAL CARE & Professionalism

As a nurse, you're trained to put others first—your patients, their families, and your team. But here's the truth: if you don't take care of yourself, you can't take care of anyone else effectively. Nursing is a demanding career, both physically and emotionally, and neglecting your own well-being can lead to burnout, stress, and even mistakes at work. On top of that, maintaining professionalism in your appearance, education, and behavior is just as important as providing quality care.

This chapter focuses on finding that delicate balance between personal care and professional responsibilities so you can thrive in your career while still prioritizing your health and happiness.

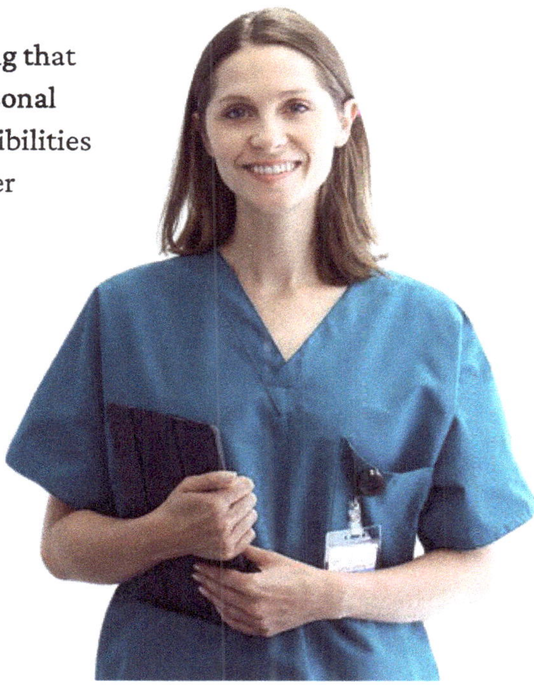

Neglecting Self-Care and Mental Health

You've probably heard the saying, "You can't pour from an empty cup." As a nurse, this couldn't be more true. Long shifts, emotional patient interactions, and constant multitasking can drain you mentally, physically, and emotionally. Many new nurses make the mistake of ignoring their own needs, thinking they're "too busy" or "it's selfish to take a break." But here's the reality: self-care isn't selfish; it's necessary.

How to Prioritize Self-Care:

- **Schedule time for yourself.** Even on busy days, take five to ten minutes to step away, breathe deeply, and reset.
- **Practice healthy habits.** Drink plenty of water during your shift, pack nutritious snacks, and aim for regular sleep when you're off.
- **Seek support when needed.** If you're feeling overwhelmed, don't hesitate to reach out to trusted colleagues, mentors, or even a counselor. Taking care of your mental health is just as important as physical well-being.

By taking care of yourself, you're not only improving your ability to care for others but also setting a positive example for your colleagues.

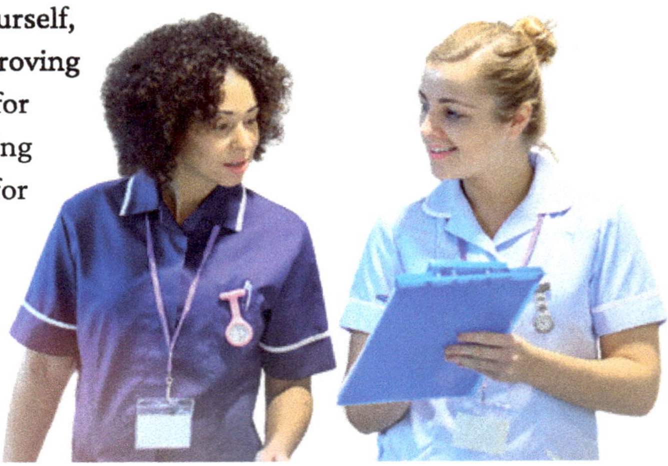

Not Maintaining a Professional Appearance

You've made it through nursing school, passed your boards, and landed your first job. But how you present yourself on the job speaks volumes about your professionalism. Maintaining a clean, polished appearance not only inspires trust from your patients but also shows respect for your workplace and the profession as a whole.

Why Appearance Matters:

- Patients and families often form first impressions within seconds. A neat, professional look can help them feel more confident in your abilities.
- Your colleagues and supervisors are more likely to view you as dependable and serious about your work.

Tips for a Professional Look:

- Keep your scrubs clean, wrinkle-free, and properly fitted.
- Wear comfortable yet professional shoes that are safe and supportive.
- Pay attention to hygiene—trimmed nails, clean hair, and minimal jewelry are typically part of workplace policies.

Professionalism isn't about being flashy—it's about showing that you respect the role you're in and the people you serve.

Failing to Keep Up with Continuing Education Requirements

Nursing is a constantly evolving field. New research, updated guidelines, and innovative technologies mean that what you learned in nursing school will only take you so far. Staying current with continuing education (CE) requirements is not just about keeping your license—it's about staying at the top of your game as a nurse.

Why Continuing Education Matters:

- It ensures you're providing evidence-based, up-to-date care to your patients.
- It helps you stay confident and competent as your career progresses.
- It can open doors for career advancement and specialization.

How to Stay on Top of CE Requirements:

- Sign up for alerts from your state board of nursing so you're always aware of deadlines.
- Take advantage of online CE courses or in-person workshops offered by your employer.
- Don't wait until the last minute—spread out your learning over the year so it's manageable.

Being proactive about your education shows dedication to your role and helps you grow into the best nurse you can be.

Ignoring Work-Life Balance

It's easy to get caught up in the grind of nursing, especially when you're new. Long shifts, overtime, and the emotional weight of patient care can make it feel like your work is your whole life. But ignoring your personal life and failing to recharge will lead to burnout—and burnout is a fast track to losing your passion for nursing.

Signs of Burnout to Watch For:

- Constant exhaustion, even on your days off
- Feeling detached from your work or patients
- Difficulty concentrating or making decisions
- Frequent irritability or frustration

Strategies for Work-Life Balance:

- **Set boundaries.** It's okay to say no to extra shifts if you're feeling drained.
- **Find activities outside of work.** Hobbies, exercise, or spending time with loved ones can help you recharge.
- **Unplug from work.** Leave work at work—mentally and physically. Avoid checking emails or thinking about tasks when you're off.
- **Prioritize rest.** You can't give your best to others if you're constantly running on empty.

Work-life balance isn't a luxury; it's a necessity. By taking time to care for yourself and maintain a fulfilling personal life, you'll be better equipped to handle the demands of your nursing career.

Personal care and professionalism go hand in hand. When you take care of yourself—physically, emotionally, and mentally—you show up as your best self for your patients, your colleagues, and your career. Nursing is a journey, and the habits you build now will sustain you for years to come. So, take a deep breath, invest in yourself, and know that by prioritizing both personal care and professionalism, you're setting the stage for a long and rewarding career.

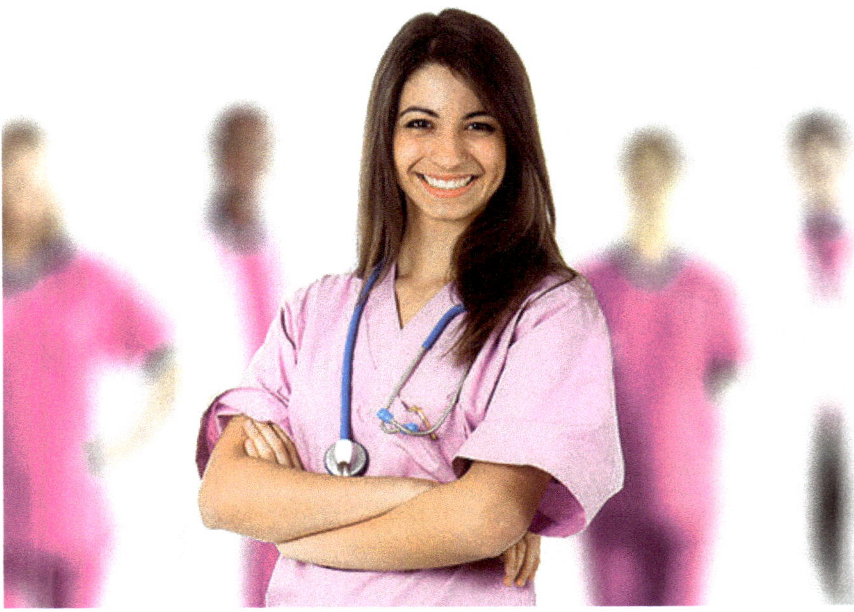

Chapter **Thirteen**

MEDICATION & Treatment Errors

Administering medications and performing treatments are core responsibilities in nursing, but they're also areas where mistakes can have life-altering consequences. As a new nurse, it's easy to feel the pressure of managing complex medication regimens and treatments, especially when working in fast-paced environments. However, slowing down and double-checking your work can make all the difference in keeping your patients safe.

This chapter dives into some of the most common medication and treatment errors, explaining how they happen and how to avoid them. With the right approach and attention to detail, you'll develop habits that will keep your patients safe and give you peace of mind.

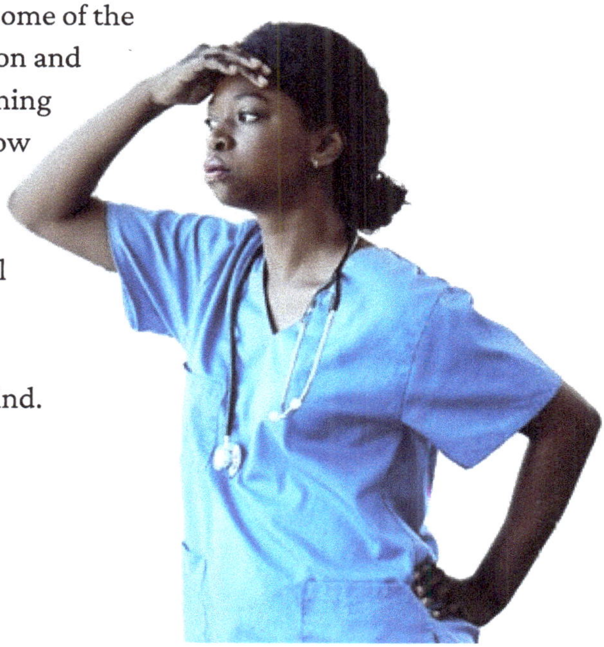

Administering Medications Without Understanding Their Purpose

It's not enough to know the name of a medication or the dose to administer. You also need to understand why the medication is being given. Every drug has a purpose, and knowing it helps you anticipate its effects, potential side effects, and how it fits into the patient's overall treatment plan.

For example, if a patient is prescribed furosemide (a diuretic), you'll expect increased urination as a normal effect. However, if they suddenly develop dangerously low blood pressure, you'll understand how the medication might have contributed and take appropriate action.

How to Avoid This Mistake:

- Take a moment to review the purpose of each medication before administering it. If you don't know why a patient is receiving a specific drug, don't be afraid to ask a colleague or look it up.
- Use resources like drug guides, online references, or your hospital's pharmacist to fill in gaps in your knowledge.

Remember, asking questions shows that you care about patient safety—not knowing and proceeding anyway is where the danger lies.

Failing to Check for Drug Allergies

Before administering any medication, it's critical to confirm whether your patient has any known drug allergies. This step might seem obvious, but in the rush of a busy shift, it's a mistake that can slip through the cracks. Administering a drug to someone with an allergy can result in anything from a mild rash to a life-threatening anaphylactic reaction.

How to Avoid This Mistake:

- Always check the patient's allergy status during your initial assessment and confirm it again before giving any medications.
- If you're unsure, double-check the patient's medical record and, when in doubt, ask the patient directly.
- Be vigilant when administering medications with common allergens, such as antibiotics like penicillin.

Never assume the information in the chart is 100% accurate—patients' allergy statuses can change, or records may have been entered incorrectly.

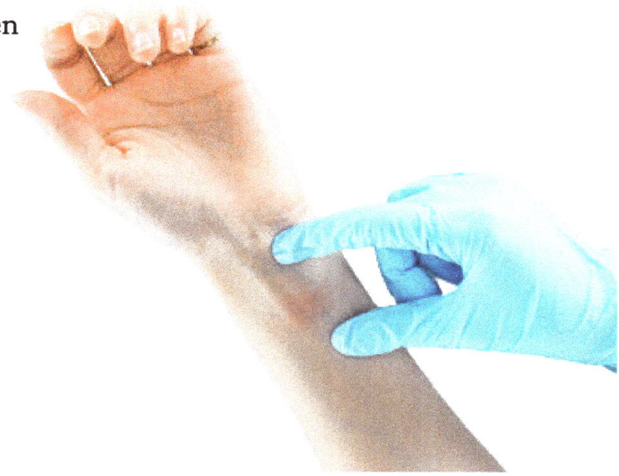

Improper Use of Infusion Pumps

Infusion pumps are powerful tools that make delivering IV medications and fluids more precise, but they're only as reliable as the person programming them. Incorrect settings, like administering the wrong flow rate, can lead to underdosing or overdosing your patient.

For instance, if you set a pump to deliver medication over 15 minutes instead of an hour, it could lead to dangerous side effects or complications.

How to Avoid This Mistake:

- Take the time to learn how your facility's infusion pumps work, including their settings and alarm systems.
- Always double-check the rate, dose, and timing before starting an infusion. If you're unsure, ask a colleague or supervisor for help.
- Follow your facility's protocols for programming pumps and verify calculations if needed.

Skipping the "Flush" Between IV Medications

Administering multiple medications through the same IV line without properly flushing it in between can lead to medication incompatibilities. Some medications can react with each other, forming precipitates that could clog the IV line or, worse, harm the patient.

For example, combining calcium and ceftriaxone without flushing can result in a life-threatening precipitate in the bloodstream.

How to Avoid This Mistake:

- Always flush the IV line with normal saline (or the appropriate solution) before and after administering medications, unless otherwise specified.
- Use drug compatibility charts to verify whether medications can safely be administered together.

Taking this extra step may seem tedious, but it's essential for ensuring the safety and efficacy of the medications you're administering.

Medication and treatment errors can feel intimidating, but they're also some of the easiest mistakes to prevent if you slow down, stay vigilant, and never stop learning. Each dose you administer and each treatment you perform is an opportunity to provide safe, excellent care—and with practice, these habits will become second nature. Always remember, it's better to ask for clarification or take a few extra minutes than to risk compromising your patient's safety.

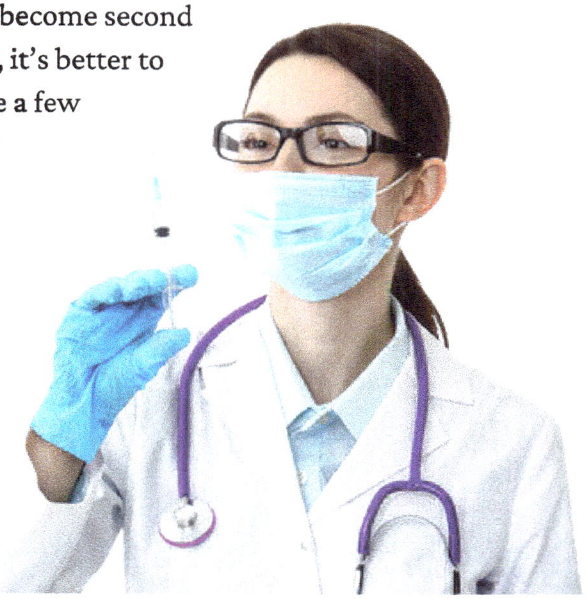

Chapter **Fourteen**

MISTAKES IN Safety Protocol

Patient safety is one of your top priorities as a nurse, but in the hustle and bustle of a busy shift, it's easy to overlook small details. Unfortunately, those small details can have big consequences. Forgetting to follow safety protocols doesn't just put your patients at risk—it can endanger you, your colleagues, and even other patients.

This chapter focuses on common safety protocol mistakes that new nurses often make and provides practical tips to help you avoid them. By building these habits early in your career, you'll create a safer environment for everyone and feel more confident in your ability to handle high-pressure situations.

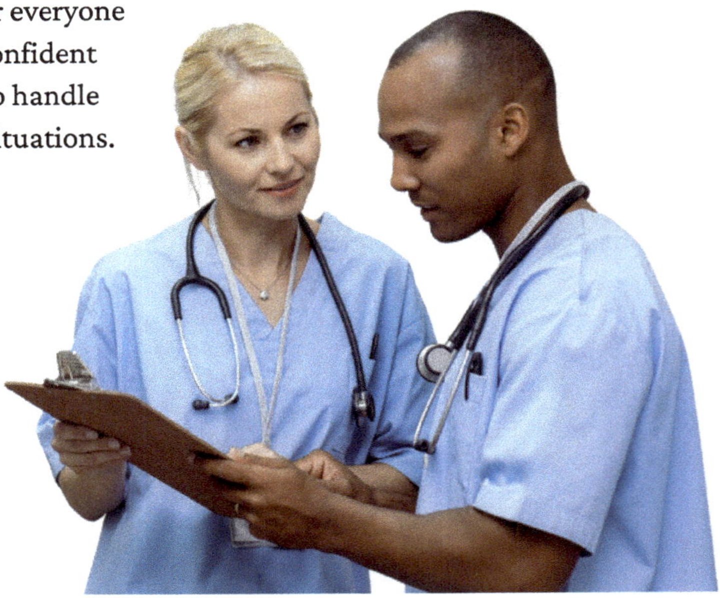

Forgetting to Activate Bed Alarms for Fall-Risk Patients

Falls are one of the most common—and preventable—safety incidents in healthcare settings. Patients who are weak, confused, or recovering from surgery are often at high risk of falling. Bed alarms are a simple yet effective tool for alerting staff when these patients attempt to get up without assistance. However, one common mistake is forgetting to activate these alarms after repositioning a patient or setting up their bed.

To prevent falls, make it a habit to assess your patients' fall risk at the beginning of your shift and ensure bed and chair alarms are activated as needed. Also, educate patients and their families on the importance of calling for help before getting up. This small step can prevent serious injuries and costly complications.

Failing to Follow Isolation Precautions

Isolation precautions exist for a reason: to protect patients, staff, and visitors from the spread of infectious diseases. Whether it's a patient with Clostridioides difficile (C. diff) requiring contact precautions or someone with airborne-transmissible tuberculosis, skipping these protocols—even just once—can have severe consequences.

Common mistakes include forgetting to wear the appropriate personal protective equipment (PPE), not performing proper hand hygiene when entering or leaving an isolation room, or failing to dispose of contaminated materials correctly.

How to Avoid This Mistake:

- Familiarize yourself with the types of isolation precautions (contact, droplet, airborne) and what each requires.
- Always check isolation signage before entering a patient's room.
- If you're unsure, ask a colleague or check your facility's infection control policy.

Remember, these precautions aren't just about protecting the patient—they're about protecting you and everyone else in the facility.

Improper Disposal of Sharps and Hazardous Materials

It might seem like a small thing, but improper disposal of sharps (like needles) and hazardous materials can lead to injuries, infections, and fines from regulatory agencies. You've probably heard this rule a thousand times: "Never recap a used needle." But in the rush of a busy shift, it can be tempting to take shortcuts, like tossing a needle into a regular trash bin or recapping it quickly "just this once."

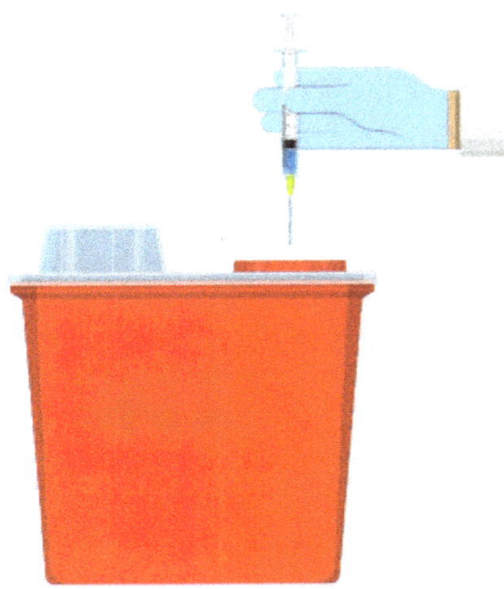

These shortcuts are never worth the risk. Recapping needles or disposing of sharps improperly can cause accidental needle sticks, exposing you or others to bloodborne pathogens. Similarly, failing to dispose of hazardous materials, such as chemotherapy drugs or body fluids, according to OSHA and facility guidelines can pose risks to the entire staff.

How to Avoid This Mistake:

- Always place used sharps immediately into designated sharps containers. Never recap needles.
- Follow your facility's protocols for disposing of hazardous materials. If you're unsure, ask your supervisor or consult the policies.
- Be mindful of sharps container fill levels—never force a sharp into an overfilled container.

By committing to these safety protocols, you're not just meeting regulatory requirements—you're actively creating a safer environment for your patients, your team, and yourself. Safety isn't just a policy; it's a mindset, and the habits you build now will serve you throughout your career.

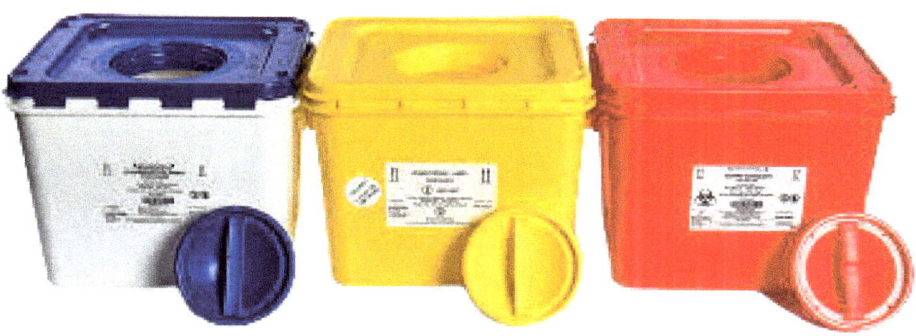

Chapter **Fifteen**

MISTAKES IN Career Growth

As a new nurse, you've already achieved something incredible: earning your degree, passing your exams, and stepping into one of the most rewarding yet challenging professions out there. But here's the thing—graduation isn't the end of your education. In fact, it's just the beginning. Nursing is a career of lifelong learning and growth. The moment you stop striving to learn, develop, and improve is the moment you stop serving your patients, your colleagues, and yourself to the best of your ability.

This chapter is all about common mistakes nurses make when it comes to their professional growth and development. Whether it's resisting feedback, ignoring career goals, or underestimating.

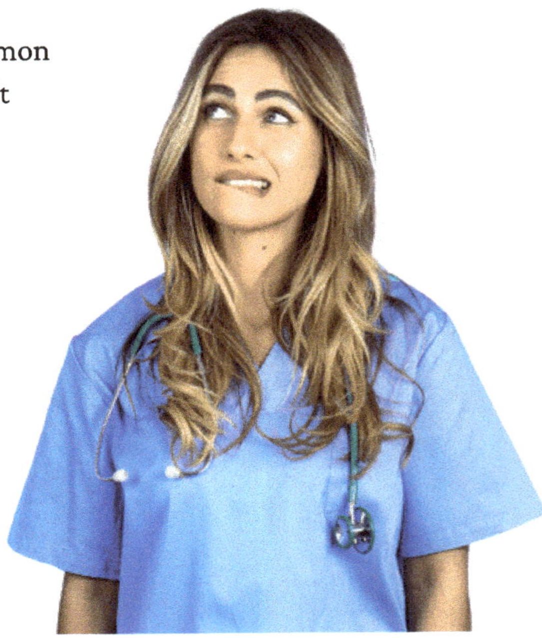

Thinking You Know It All

One of the most dangerous mistakes you can make early in your career is believing you've "learned it all" now that you've graduated and passed the NCLEX. Nursing is a dynamic, ever-changing profession. Treatments, technology, and best practices evolve constantly, and staying humble and open to learning is essential for success.

Instead of feeling like you need to know everything right away, embrace the mindset of a lifelong learner. Ask questions when you're unsure, seek out additional training, and stay curious. Remember, no one expects you to have all the answers immediately—it's your willingness to learn that will make you a better nurse.

Avoiding Constructive Feedback

Let's be honest: no one enjoys being told they're doing something wrong. But constructive feedback is one of the most valuable tools for your growth as a nurse. Whether it's a supervisor pointing out an error in your documentation or a colleague offering advice on patient care, feedback is an opportunity to improve—not a personal attack.

Instead of avoiding or dismissing feedback, approach it with an open mind. Ask questions to clarify how you can improve and thank the person for their input. This attitude not only helps you grow but also demonstrates professionalism and a commitment to excellence.

Not Setting Long-Term Career Goals

When you're just starting out, it's easy to focus on surviving your shifts rather than thinking about the bigger picture. But taking the time to set long-term career goals early on will give your nursing career direction and purpose. Do you see yourself specializing in pediatrics, becoming a nurse educator, or even pursuing advanced practice nursing?

Start by reflecting on your interests and strengths. Then, map out a plan for how to get there. Whether it's obtaining certifications, pursuing further education, or gaining experience in a specific area, having clear goals will keep you motivated and on track for success.

Ignoring Opportunities for Leadership Roles

Leadership might feel like something you'll worry about "later," but the truth is, leadership skills are valuable at every stage of your nursing career. Whether it's mentoring a fellow new nurse, taking charge during a crisis, or joining a committee at your facility, stepping into leadership opportunities early on can set you apart.

Leadership doesn't **always** mean managing others—**it's about** being a role model, advocating for patients, and contributing to the improvement of your workplace. Look for small ways to build

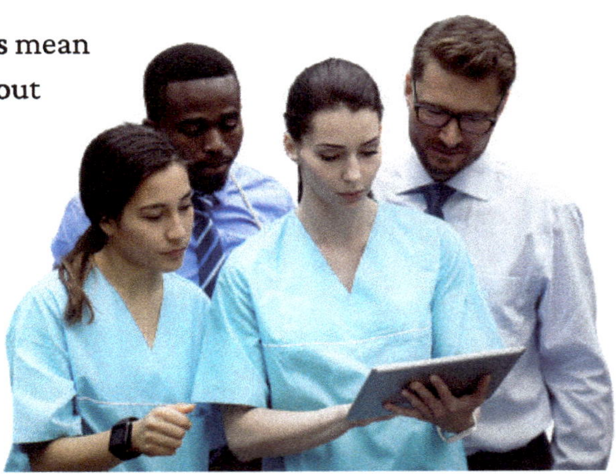

your leadership skills, and don't be afraid to volunteer for new responsibilities.

Key Takeaways for Growth and Development

- **Stay humble** and embrace learning at every stage of your career.
- View **constructive feedback** as a tool for growth, not criticism.
- Set **long-term career goals** to give your nursing journey direction.
- Seek out opportunities to **develop leadership skills** early, even in small ways.

Growth as a nurse is a never-ending process, but that's part of what makes this career so rewarding. The more you invest in your own development, the more confident, capable, and fulfilled you'll feel—not just as a nurse, but as a person.

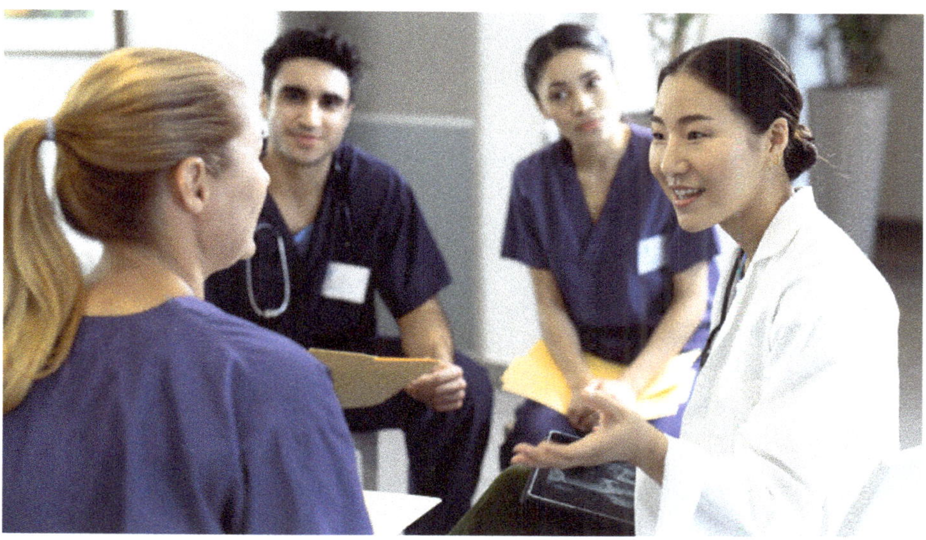

Chapter **Sixteen**

ERRORS WITH Patient Interaction

As nurses, we're often the first and last point of contact for our patients. We're their caregivers, advocates, and sometimes even their lifeline in challenging moments. But in the whirlwind of a busy shift, it's easy to fall into habits that can unintentionally make patients feel unheard, dismissed, or misunderstood. Patient interaction isn't just about completing tasks—it's about connecting with people on a human level.

This chapter focuses on the common mistakes nurses make when interacting with patients and their families. By learning to avoid these pitfalls, you'll not only provide better care but also build trust, foster rapport, and leave your patients feeling respected and valued.

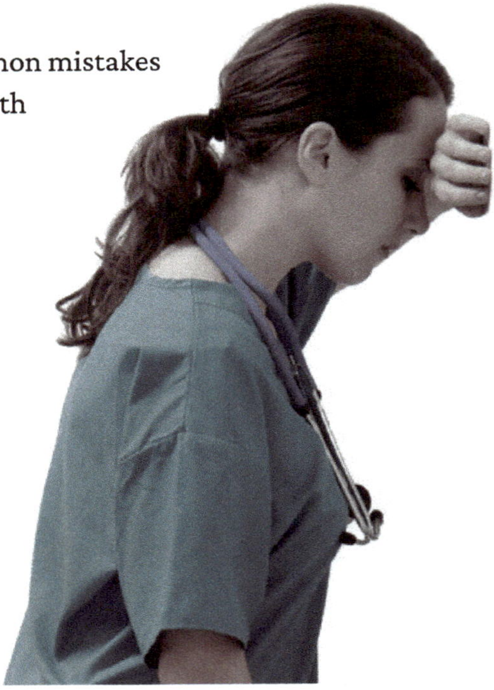

Not Actively Listening to Patients

Have you ever been in a conversation where you felt like the other person wasn't truly listening? It's frustrating, right? Now imagine feeling that way when you're scared, vulnerable, or in pain. For patients, feeling unheard can make an already stressful experience even worse.

Active listening is more than just hearing what your patients are saying —it's about fully engaging with them. Make eye contact, nod, and use verbal cues like "I understand" or "Tell me more." Even when you're pressed for time, taking a few extra moments to really listen can make a huge difference in how your patients perceive their care.

How to Avoid This Mistake:

- Eliminate distractions. Put down the chart or step away from the computer when talking to a patient.
- Paraphrase what the patient says to confirm understanding. For example: "So you're saying the pain gets worse when you move your leg. Is that correct?"
- Be patient. Sometimes patients need a moment to find the right words to express themselves.

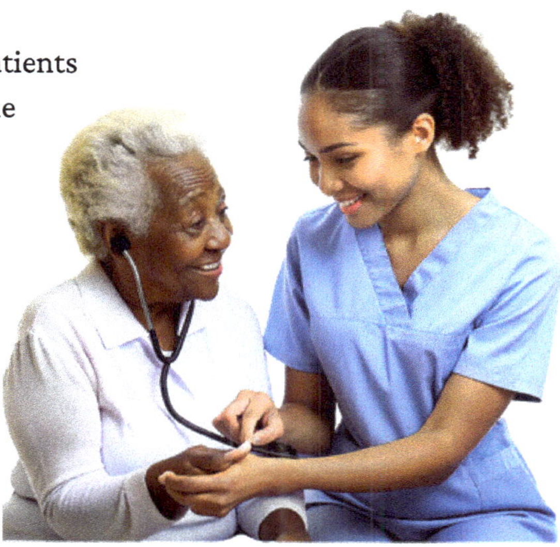

Failing to Respect Cultural Differences

Every patient comes with their own unique background, beliefs, and values, which can significantly influence how they view healthcare. A one-size-fits-all approach doesn't work in nursing, and failing to respect cultural differences can lead to misunderstandings or even harm.

For example, some cultures may have specific preferences regarding modesty, diet, or end-of-life care. As a nurse, it's your responsibility to approach these differences with respect and curiosity. You don't have to know everything about every culture, but you do need to be open to learning and willing to ask questions.

How to Avoid This Mistake:

- Use open-ended questions to understand a patient's preferences. For instance, "Is there anything about your culture or beliefs I should know to provide better care?"
- Avoid making assumptions. Just because someone belongs to a particular cultural group doesn't mean they adhere to every practice associated with it.
- Take advantage of resources like cultural competency training or language interpreters when needed.

Rushing Through Patient Interactions

Let's face it—there are days when your to-do list feels never-ending. It's tempting to rush through patient interactions to move on to the next task, but doing so can leave your patients feeling like they're just another item to check off your list. Patients notice when you're rushing, and it can damage the trust and connection you're trying to build.

Even when you're short on time, small gestures of empathy and compassion can go a long way. A warm smile, a gentle touch, or even a brief moment of genuine conversation can make your patients feel cared for and valued.

How to Avoid This Mistake:

- Prioritize quality over quantity. It's better to spend two meaningful minutes with a patient than ten rushed ones.
- Be mindful of your body language. Avoid appearing hurried or distracted, even when you're feeling the pressure.
- Use simple phrases like, "I wish I could stay longer, but I want to make sure I check on everyone. Is there anything I can do for you right now?"

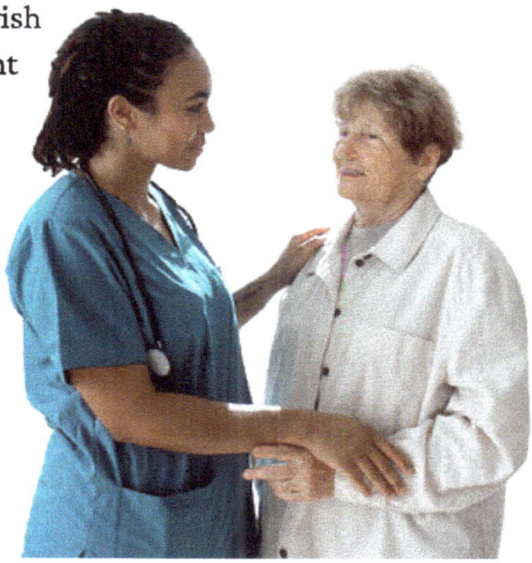

Making Promises You Can't Keep

In an effort to reassure or comfort patients, it's easy to slip into making promises you may not be able to fulfill. Saying things like, "I'll be back in five minutes" or "You'll feel better soon" might seem harmless, but if those promises aren't kept, it can erode trust and leave patients feeling disappointed or abandoned.

Instead, focus on managing expectations honestly. It's okay to say, "I'll do my best to get back to you soon," or "We'll do everything we can to help with your pain." Patients appreciate honesty, even when it's not exactly what they want to hear.

How to Avoid This Mistake:

- Be realistic about what you can deliver. Don't make commitments you can't keep.
- If you do get delayed, check back in with the patient to explain the situation. A quick update can help manage their expectations and prevent frustration.
- Communicate transparently about what you can and cannot control.

The Power of Connection

Your interactions with patients are some of the most impactful moments of their healthcare experience. By actively listening, respecting their individuality, and being present in each interaction, you can create a sense of trust and comfort that goes beyond the physical care you provide.

Mistakes in patient interaction are often unintentional, but they can have lasting effects on how patients perceive their care—and on your own satisfaction as a nurse. By focusing on building meaningful, respectful connections, you'll not only avoid these common missteps but also create a more fulfilling and rewarding nursing career.

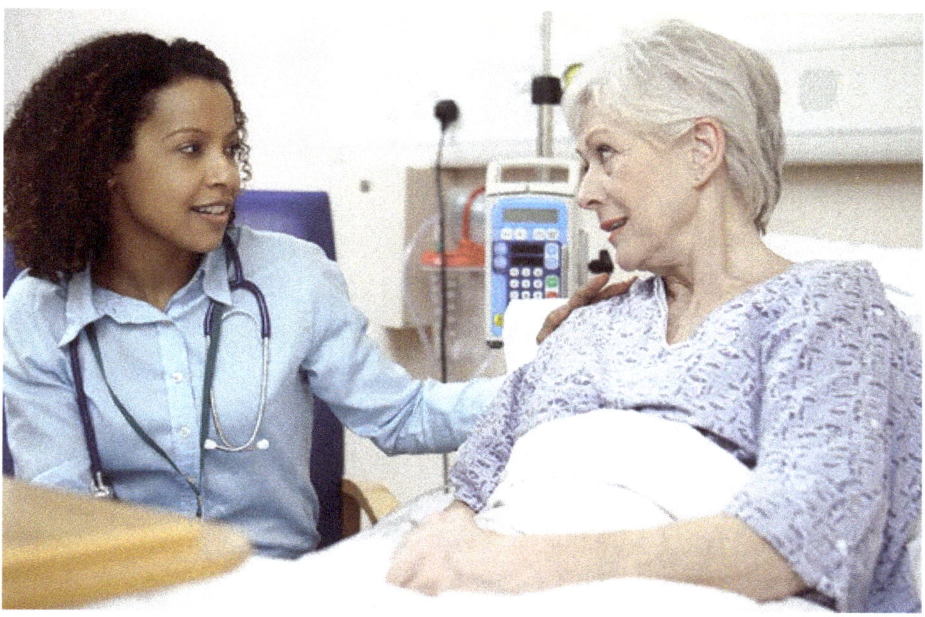

Chapter **Seventeen**

MISTAKES IN
Crisis & Emergency

In the world of nursing, emergencies are inevitable. Whether it's a patient coding, a sudden drop in vitals, or a hospital-wide crisis like a fire or disaster, being prepared for high-stress situations is part of the job. But let's face it—when you're new, emergencies can feel overwhelming. You might freeze, panic, or feel unsure about what to do next. That's normal at first, but the goal is to learn how to stay calm, act decisively, and work effectively under pressure.

This chapter explores some of the common mistakes nurses make during crises and emergencies and provides actionable tips to help you respond like a pro. The more prepared and confident.

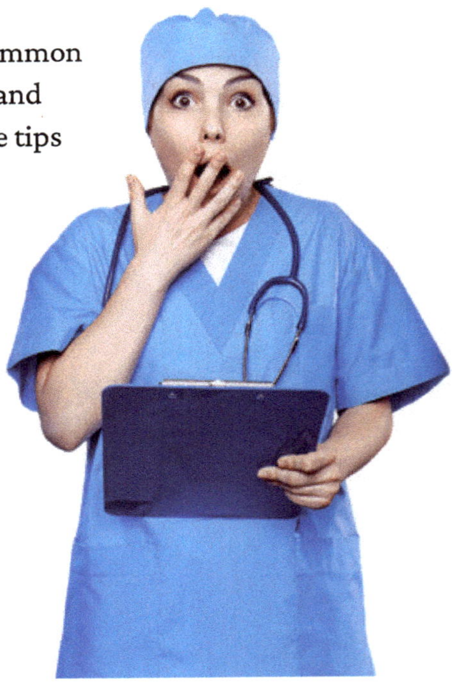

Freezing Under Pressure

It's natural to feel paralyzed in a high-stakes emergency, especially early in your career when you're still building confidence. The sudden rush of adrenaline can make it hard to think clearly or remember what you've been trained to do. But freezing under pressure doesn't help your patient, your team, or yourself.

The key to overcoming this instinct is preparation and practice. When you're well-prepared, you'll default to your training instead of panic. Take a deep breath, focus on your role in the situation, and remember that you're part of a team. You don't have to do it all yourself—you just have to stay composed and do your part.

Staying Calm and Focused in Emergencies

Staying calm during an emergency is easier said than done, but it's one of the most important skills you can develop. When chaos erupts, your demeanor can either help bring order to the situation or add to the stress. Patients, families, and even colleagues will look to you for reassurance and direction.

Here's a tip: break the situation into manageable steps. Instead of focusing on the entire crisis, ask yourself, What can I do right now to help? Whether it's starting chest compressions, calling for backup, or documenting events, focus on action over anxiety. Practicing mindfulness techniques, like deep breathing, can also help you keep a cool head in the heat of the moment.

Not Participating in Mock Drills

Mock drills might feel like a nuisance when you're already juggling a full schedule, but they're invaluable for building your emergency response skills. Whether it's a code blue simulation, a fire drill, or a mass casualty exercise, these drills give you a chance to practice in a low-stakes environment.

Skipping drills means you'll be less prepared when a real emergency strikes. Instead, treat them as an opportunity to identify gaps in your knowledge, ask questions, and refine your skills. When the real thing happens, you'll be grateful for the practice.

Preparing for Real-Life Crises Through Simulation

Many facilities offer simulation labs to help staff prepare for emergencies. These controlled environments allow you to work through scenarios like cardiac arrests or trauma situations without the pressure of real life. Don't shy away from these opportunities—they're a safe space to make mistakes, learn, and grow.

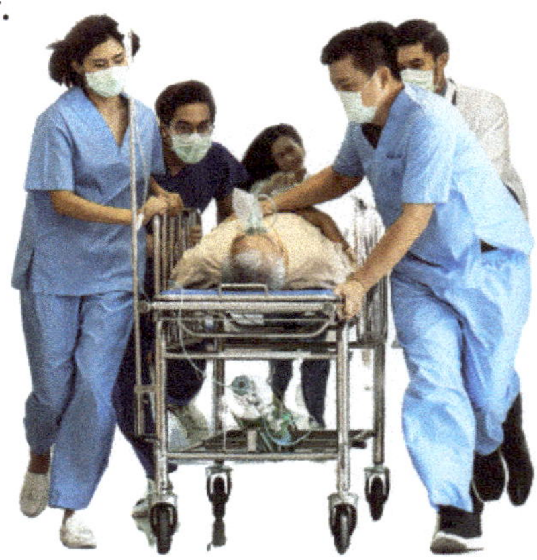

Simulations also help you build muscle memory, so when an actual emergency occurs, you can act instinctively and confidently. If your facility doesn't offer regular simulations, take the initiative to review emergency protocols and run through scenarios mentally.

Failing to Report Unsafe Practices

Speaking up when you see something unsafe can be intimidating, especially if you're new or the person at fault is more experienced than you. But keeping quiet about unsafe practices—whether it's a missed protocol, improper equipment use, or a colleague's mistake—can put patients and staff at risk.

Remember, reporting unsafe practices isn't about assigning blame; it's about protecting everyone involved. Approach the situation professionally and focus on the facts. Many facilities have anonymous reporting systems if you're uncomfortable addressing issues directly.

Speaking Up to Protect Patients and Colleagues

Advocating for your patients and colleagues is a vital part of being a nurse. If you notice something that could harm a patient—like a potential medication error or equipment malfunction—don't hesitate to speak up. Even if you're wrong, it's better to err on the side of caution than to stay silent and risk harm.

The same goes for protecting your team. If a colleague is overwhelmed or making mistakes, offer help or alert a supervisor. Nursing is a team effort, and looking out for one another is essential in high-pressure situations.

Emergencies are one of the most stressful parts of nursing, but they're also where you have the opportunity to make the greatest impact. By preparing yourself mentally and physically, practicing regularly, and learning to stay calm under pressure, you'll be ready to step up when it matters most. Remember, no nurse handles an emergency alone—you're part of a team, and together, you can rise to any challenge.

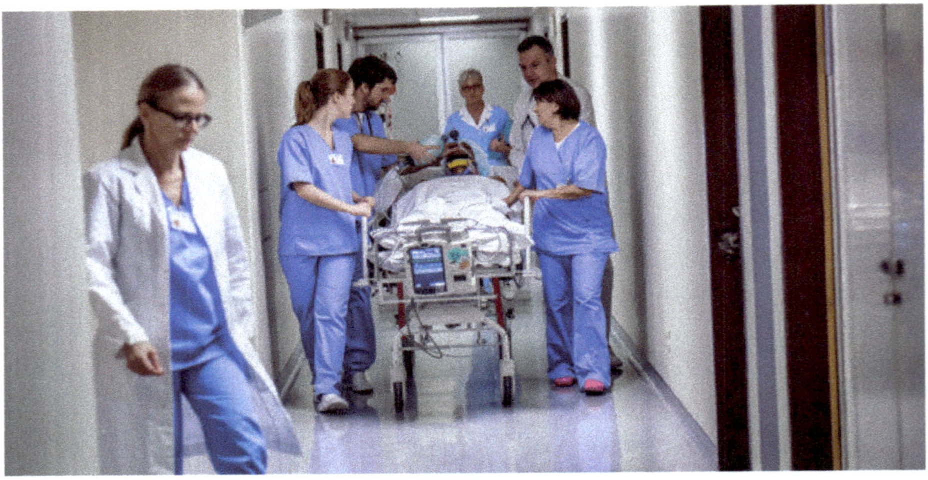

Chapter **Eighteen**

EXCELLING IN YOUR Nursing Career

Becoming a nurse is more than just starting a career—it's stepping into a calling that allows you to make a profound difference in the lives of others. But as fulfilling as nursing can be, it also comes with its share of challenges. Long shifts, emotional situations, and the fast pace of healthcare can take a toll. So how do you not just survive as a nurse, but truly thrive?

In this final chapter, we'll explore how to stay motivated, grow in your career, and leave a lasting impact in the field of nursing. Whether you're just starting out or envisioning where you'll be in 10 years, these tips will...

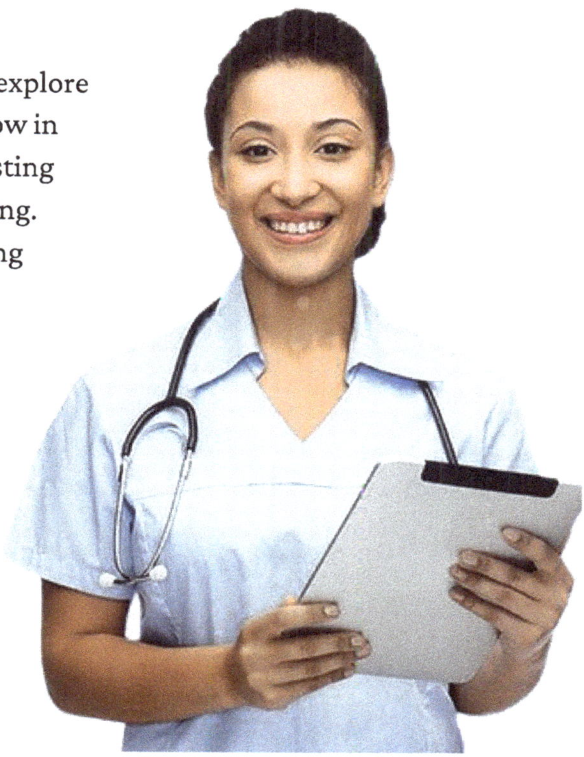

Staying Motivated in Your Career

Nursing is a rewarding yet demanding profession, and staying motivated can feel like a challenge after long shifts or during difficult days. It's important to reconnect regularly with why you chose nursing in the first place. Was it the opportunity to care for others? The chance to make a tangible difference? Whatever your reason, holding onto that purpose will help you push through the tough times.

Celebrate the small victories—those moments when a patient says "thank you," when you comfort a worried family member, or when you see measurable improvement in a patient's health. These moments are what make nursing so impactful, and taking time to...

Exploring Specializations & Advanced Practice

One of the most exciting things about nursing is the endless opportunities for growth. As you gain experience, you may find that certain areas of nursing speak to your interests and passions. Whether it's working in pediatrics, oncology, critical care, mental health, or even becoming a nurse educator, there are countless pathways to explore.

If you're not sure where to start, reflect on the types of patients or cases that energize you the most. Do you enjoy the fast-paced environment of an ER? Or do you prefer the one-on-one connections in home health care? As you explore these options, consider taking additional certifications, shadowing colleagues in different specialties, or pursuing advanced degrees, such as becoming a Nurse Practitioner (NP) or Clinical Nurse Specialist (CNS).

Specializing not only deepens your skills but also opens doors to leadership roles, increased earning potential, and opportunities to create a more significant impact. Keep an open mind—sometimes, the area you least expect to love becomes the one you can't imagine leaving.

Building a Legacy of Excellence in Nursing

Thriving as a nurse means more than just excelling at your day-to-day responsibilities—it's about creating a lasting impact on your patients, colleagues, and the profession itself. Think of every shift as an opportunity to build your legacy of excellence.

How do you do this? By consistently showing kindness, compassion, and dedication. By mentoring newer nurses and sharing the lessons you've learned. By advocating for patients and making their voices heard. And by always striving for improvement in your practice.

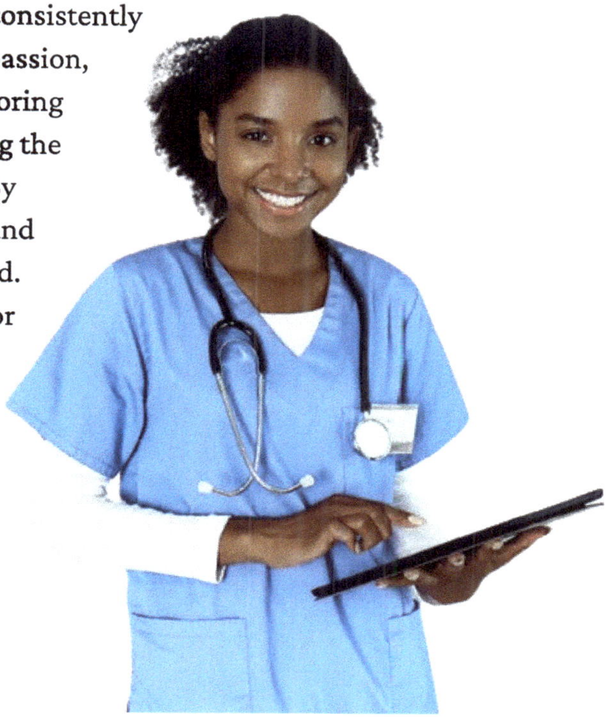

Remember, nursing isn't just a job—it's a legacy you leave with every patient you care for and every colleague you uplift. When you look back on your career, what kind of difference will you want to have made? By focusing on your growth, maintaining your motivation, and embracing opportunities for advancement, you'll not only thrive in your career but inspire others to do the same.

Final Thoughts

Thriving as a nurse isn't about perfection—it's about passion, persistence, and progress. You will make mistakes, face challenges, and have days that feel overwhelming. But you will also experience incredible rewards: saving lives, bringing comfort to others, and growing both personally and professionally.

Take care of yourself, embrace every learning opportunity, and stay connected to the reason you became a nurse in the first place. Whether you're just starting out or looking to build the next chapter of your career, the possibilities are limitless. Nursing is a journey, and you're writing your story every day. Make it one you're proud of.

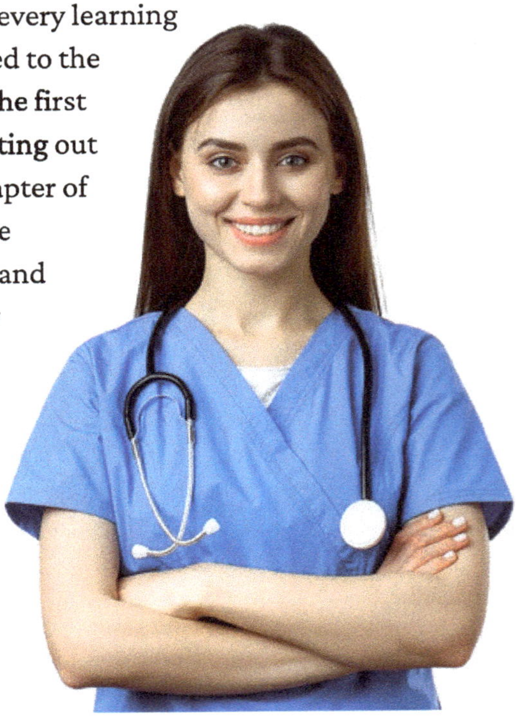